Sciatica Exercises

*Simple Techniques, Stretching And Yoga Exercises To Find
Relief From Back Pain And Sciatica. Recover Your Life Forever
Without Drugs Or Surgery*

William M Wittman

Table Of Contents

CHAPTER ONE

☙

Understanding sciatica

The definition of sciatica identifies outward symptoms originating out of the peripheral nerve, that's the huge nerve generated from several large nerves which branch away from every side of the low spinal column. The nerves proceed through the entire buttock area on each side and continue down the back of each leg. Below the knee, then the plantar nerve divides in to two branches which proceed the leg into the foot and ankle. However, many people today telephone outward symptoms any place in the leg, authentic thoracic symptoms happen at the buttock area and might stretch the back part of the thigh and back to the upper leg and feet. Broadly speaking, the further bloated the guts is, the farther the indicators will probably expand the leg down. When you'll find rare neurological disorders, which could cause the progression of sciatica as a result of lead nerve pathology, in the majority of cases sciatica can be really a symptom of several other underlying problem. Even the most prevalent causes of sciatica could be simplified in to two major categories, nerve wracking and muscular contraction. Nerve compression may be a consequence of various causes, however it's most frequently due to a bulge or insertion of a couple of intervertebral disks in the low thoracic spinal column.

Sciatica is pain at the back or hip that radiates on to the buttock and back of the leg across the sciatic nerve, usually to the foot. Each nerve transmits signals for motor controller of several muscles at the leg in addition to sensation towards the leg. The pain generated is resulting from an affected or inflamed gastrointestinal tract wracking and may appear after a personal accident, muscular stress, or herniated disc that presses on the guts.

Which exactly are the outward indicators?

The pain of sciatica usually takes quite a few forms - it can seem as a cramp in the leg, pain up on sitting, pain along with coughing or sneezing, and could arrive as tingling, tingling, burning, electric jolt such as sensation or as "pinsand needles" across the leg. The pain often occurs on a single side. Many individuals have sharp pain in 1 area of their hip or leg and numbness in different pieces. The senses might also be felt over the back of the calf or over the sole of their foot. Muscle fatigue may happen due to pressure or pain on the guts.

The pain often begins slowly and progressively becoming worse; definite activities can commence the observable symptoms for example;

Sitting or standing for extended intervals

At nighttime

When coughing, coughing, or laughing

When bending backward or walking than a couple of yards, particularly if due to spinal stenosis

Which exactly are the causes?

The sciatic nerves are the longest nerves in your system, running out of the lower back down the buttock and cool, and continuing down the back part of every leg entirely into the foot. Each carry neural signals for motor controller of several muscles from the leg in addition to sensation towards the leg.

Such a thing that combats a sciatic nerve for prolonged amounts of time could lead to sciatica. Sometimes this is caused by a ruptured disk in the low spine. In case the disk ruptures, their inner linking substance can float and shove against nerves. Age-related modifications to the backbone induce degeneration of these disks and also the vertebral tissues. Intervertebral discs make space between your bones, so allowing a location for those nerves to maneuver while they leave the back. Degeneration of these vertebrae may give rise to a narrowing of the distance between nerves which make a difference to a nerve root that induces similar signs.

Traumatization out of an auto crash or blow into the backbone may harm the sciatic nerve right away, because may muscle breeds of this lower back muscles and nerves of the piriformis muscle which runs directly across the guts. Since these muscles act as tight or move into anxiety, they are able to cause a rope-like strain which disturbs the nerve.

In addition to growing older, being at work which demands constant twisting, heavy lifting or forcing may make you likely to sciatica. The sitting which does occur as a consequence of a desk-job or being too sedentary may additionally put extra strain on the back and legs.

Evidence and tests

Sciatica may possibly be shown by way of a neurological and orthopedic study of their spine and thighs. Pain down the leg might be duplicated by lifting your leg straight off the table. Tests are guided by the suspected cause of this disorder, according to the history, symptoms, and pattern of symptom improvement.

Under ordinary conditions, there's loads of space around the spinal cord nerves by which they branch off from the back and then leave the spine (technically, the cervical back finishes at the middle thoracic spinal column and becomes a package of different nerves called the cauda equina at the low lumbers, however for the interest of simplicity, then i will be speaking about it since the back). However, the opening at which the nerve exits the spine may get substituted by a couple of stuff, leading to compression and irritation of the nerves. Probably one of the very typical sources of neural compression is that a disk bulge, that can also be referred to as a disk herniation, or disk protrusion. The disks have a outer cartilage wall and also are full of a gel-like material that offers the spine with numerous angles of freedom and shock-absorption. The wall may get damaged (in a sense which are going to probably be discussed later) and the inner pressure of the gel makes it bulge out at the tip of damage. On account of the arrangement of their spine, and owing to the activities and postures which we typically participate in, disks have a tendency to bulge backward towards the back and nerves.

The huge vast majority of disk injuries are emptied or protrusions and may usually be effectively treated with the strategy which may be discussed within this publication. Disc ruptures (extrusions) tend to be somewhat more severe and may frequently require operation to attain long-term aid of symptoms. Incidentally, the definition of "ruptured disc" usually gets used wrongly (by health practitioners) to explain what's obviously a disk bulge (herniation or protrusion), and thus do not assume you will require operation if you're told there is a ruptured disc and soon you've got confirmation (in an mri or ct scanning) that the disk remains actually pliable (the provisions "extruded" or "sequestered" may show up on the imaging accounts in reference to a couple of disks) and never merely bulging or protruding. Along with disk lumps and ruptures, the distance around the spinal nerves are usually narrowed by fluctuations inside the spine associated with rheumatoid arthritis. With rheumatoid arthritis, the disks may frequently eliminate fluid and eventually become slimmer, bone fractures can thicken or shape spurs, and spinal nerves can inhale (from the bones becoming closer together) or become thicker -- each one which might narrow down the openings that the nerves pass through.

To locate the treatment for sciatica you first need to begin understanding its own nature. This appears to be an extremely straightforward job but there several individuals who translate sciatica because of a easy straight back issue. But, it's different in contrast to a normal back ache. Sciatica is clarified to be a piercing kind of headache along with electric shocks and shocks. That really is by the inflammation which starts in the plantar nerve. The sciatic nerve is the major nerve which conducts sensory purposes by the decreased spine entirely down to the feet.

The function of the sciatic nerve from the body is very essential as it's in charge of relaying information to the mind. It's accountable for organizing movement controller and sensory feedback of their feet and legs. There are lots of probable causes of the beginning of sciatica. The most prevalent disease is called a herniated spinal disk. The disk functions as a cushion into the back vertebra. But in the event the disk slides from its original location, it occupies the space for the nerves. Insulin begins, also sciatica develops. Other cases of illnesses that activate sciatica are piriformis syndrome and spinal stenosis.

The treatment for sciatica isn't exactly the exact same for several sufferers. Sciatica can be a symptom of an underlying origin. Step one towards a laughter treatment is discovering the particular condition. Consult a seasoned doctor regarding sciatica.

Establishing a highly efficient cure will start with a full medical history test, accompanied closely by clinical exams such as an Xray. These evaluations are given only in the event the physician deems them to be mandatory.

To heal sciatica is always to cover the inflammation. Medical professionals urge simple bed rest and avoiding strenuous pursuits. Medicines for anti-inflammatory and muscular relaxing purposes tend to be prescribed to the individual. In acute cases of oral steroids for a much more competitive dose of anti-inflammation are also prescribed. Patients can also go for an epidural steroid injection. This can become an immediate anti remedy for sciatica. Some traditional sufferers of sciatica prefer ice and heat packs application to the bloated area to treat the pain.

Addressing the inflammation and pain are partial remedies of sciatica. Many caregivers encourage patients to run carefully constructed exercises mixed in using physical therapy sessions. This will assist in preventing future swelling episodes.

A surgical process for the treatment cure is most likely the last alternative for patients. In lots of instances, medical procedures is unnecessary. But, it ought to be seriously contemplated when puberty isn't treated after around a few weeks of subsequent nonsurgical cure approaches.

Sciatica operation intends in order to steer clear of compression, hence providing the regular distance for the thoracic nerve to work normally. The physician might want to clean a bone surrounding the guts or eliminate a broken disk. Luckily, a fantastic proportion of folks are wholly healed from sciatica without having to undergo operation. All these are the individuals whose plantar nerves aren't injured forever. Enough timeframe to treat pain will be in 3 months to a few months for a lot of cases. Sciatica at a mild or moderate form isn't regarded as a health emergency however also the distress and pain it attracts may disturb some body from living a regular living. Hence, the best choice is to look for the help of your physician once you've the earliest signs of sciatica and learn as far as possible regarding the treatment choices which are best for you personally.

Sciatica is an indication of an accident or disease that's affecting the plantar nerve at the leg. The sciatic nerve can be found from the decreased backbone throughout the thighs, also is a significant muscle for having the capability to maneuver and texture pieces of one's own leg, commanding all it. Sciatica is made up of pain, tingling, fatigue and also tingling at the leg. But these signs may fluctuate widely in many individuals.

Which exactly are the indicators of sciatica?

As said, sciatica could be experienced in a number of diverse ways. A few accounts that a pain that is dull, but some report mild numbness, or perhaps a burning pain. The pain is usually localized to a single side of their human body and the individual can experience it just 1 leg or one among her or his spine. These symptoms may worsen when standing up unexpectedly, at that nighttime, when vibration from laughing or alternative pursuits along with later long walks and physical exercise.

So, what can I really do concern sciatica?

Take part doing press ups, this will aim the principal nuisance are as within sciatica, the buttocks, the thighs and the spine side. Extension exercises are a more low-impact means to be certain you are perhaps not in pain after. For those who have use of some pool, then ask your personal doctor concerning water exercises, that is a excellent, painless approach to get started establishing your own strength. Hamstring exercises are fantastic for handling lower back pain.

Hamstring work-outs

There are some powerful exercises for strengthening your mind. Lying leg curls - it's called hamstring curl. You want to lie to your hamstring machine on tummy whilst setting the leg curl bar all on your knees. You want to launch it then repeat it to get a long time. Great mornings - you ought to set a barbell on your shoulders while keeping your legs inflexible at position. You want to bend forwards slightly, however, the mind ought to be upwards. You've got to create your torso parallel to the ground floor. Repeat it many times.

As a result of the disposition of sciatica, there may be an inherent problem which a health care provider should tackle. Exercise can be a superb solution to diminish painful senses and boost freedom. It's actually vital that you exercise to handle the pain, as it strengthens your muscles, providing more aid, and also perhaps not only does it reduce strain, it will also allow you to prevent it later on. You need to speak to your health care provider prior to getting involved in any strenuous training.

A variety of distress are advocated by a lady who's pregnant. The cause for this may be that the climbing weight that puts strain on the rear part and thighs. Few woman additionally undergo thoracic nerve pain throughout the time period. Occurrence with the could cause extreme debilitating from the normal uneasy disquiet. The sciatica nerve may be the largest nerve in your human body that stimulates and regulates the movement of their lesser portion of their human anatomy. Whenever there's swelling and compression found from the body, pressing activity pressures the thoracic nerve resulting in severe pain.

Women who complain of thoracic nerve pain that's sharp and popping the back part of the thighs, have undergone exactly the same before maternity. Some of the chief explanations for occurrence of this pain is protracted focusing in their toes and excess weight reduction. The perfect method to decrease the pain will be always to lay to among those negative. This specific posture lowers the total weight in the back along with your thighs. Depending on the character of tasks which can be performed in day to day existence, an individual has to set postures so. This measure reduces the maturation of sciatica and decreases the pain at the back and leg.

Sciatica nerve pain may be lowered by giving warmth into your system. Usage of hot compresses, a hot tub and also a restricted temperature at the room will avert the bitterness of annoyance. It's always recommended to not make use of heels throughout pregnancy since they induce discomfort and boost the degree of sciatica. Usage of comfortable shoes with soft feet is much more preferable since they feature nil or diminished stress growth in the foot. Routine exercises will reduce the quantity of stress developed from the low back section of the human anatomy.

It really is additionally crucial to seek advice from a health care provider for approval to perform certain exercises to avoid overtraining nerve pain. Swimming is among the most useful available exercises which stop the maturation of sciatica. Pregnant woman may also look forwards for rectal yoga which provides increased rest by the worries and increases the sum of relaxation. When the pain is more bothersome, an individual has to stop by a physical therapist who'll offer help by embracing special exercises which may enhance the potency from the elements of abdomen, spine and abdominal muscles. Sciatica occurs because of temporary disorder when pregnant and will be over come little preventative steps.

Where does the pain come out?

Sciatica anxiety is pain which elicits from the reduced part of their human body due to a issue with the peripheral nerve. Many times, that is from a lumbar disc herniation which moves down on the guts. But, pinched nerves, nerve wracking, inflammation, muscular issues, injuries, or germs may be the main reason.

Can be sciatica a significant problem?

Sometimes the pain which results in sciatica are able to keep people from contributing their lives for days and sometimes maybe weeks, also could be painful at a few cases.

Sciatic nerve issues may lead to pain, a sense of tingling, soothes tingles, and burning sensations at the reduced back off to the thigh. If the signs and symptoms are intense, they are able to interfere with the ability to walk or proceed at the midsection area. Anxiety relief for back pain can be potential, however it isn't just a challenge which may be mended immediately.

Can it be crucial to find a physician?

Should you suspect you have sciatic nerve difficulties, visit your personal doctor. He'll examine your health history and provide you with a detailed examination to establish what the issue is. Fixing the underlying problems could reduce recurrences of coronary artery pain. You may well be asked to get some evaluations such as for example x-rays, MRI scans, and scans, or even electromyogram. Don't try to diagnose or cure yourself. *

So, what exactly can be done to halt the pain?

From the ago, bedrest has been certainly one of the principal treatments for sciatica. Recent studies demonstrate that bed rest is really not the most suitable choice. Bed remainder prevents you out of proceeding, and movement is obviously valuable. Various other kinds of therapy that can help with pain relief and reduce inflammation may be· exercising by extending

Your doctor may provide you a set of pain-relieving stretching. Once the pain has improved, in case you carry on using those stretches, then they are able to cut the odds of pain killers at the foreseeable future. Strengthening muscles to boost your posture can be a fantastic means to decrease the prospect of gastric pain coming back again.

Surgical processes

There are distinct kinds of operation which may help alleviate gastrointestinal pain. But, operation is a really aggressive treatment that's most frequently utilized in chronic scenarios.

Infection direction

Infection management experts will assist you to handle continuing pain difficulties. These professionals make use of various techniques depending on the intensity of one's situation. Treatment may involve medication, physical therapy or topical software or emotional therapy.

in case you believe you're experiencing the signs and symptoms of sciatic nerve pain, so you need to contact your primary care doctor when you can explore all your treatment choices.

Every person differs therefore every individual's treatment plans will probably differ. Chronic pain is never a standard condition. There are tons of options outside there which may assist you in getting on with a balanced and regular daily life.

CHAPTER TWO

❦

Degenerative bone and ligament thickening

Degenerative changes from the backbone most frequently influence the trunk portion of their spinal openings, whilst disk lumps and ruptures usually narrow front of their spinal pockets. Oftentimes, there's a level of narrowing from the disk protrusion and degenerative alterations. Additionally, further nerve wracking frequently results in swelling as a result of inflammation that's set off by disk damage or degenerative arthritis. While nerve wracking may also lead from spinal and pancreatic ailments that require operative therapy, the vast majority of instances of nerve wracking are caused by a mix of disk bulging, degenerative alterations, or inflammatory swelling and may usually be efficiently handled with the remedies mentioned in this publication. The other big group of reasons for sciatica symptoms is muscular contraction. Several muscles could lead to pain down the leg but merely a single muscle really meets the indicators of authentic sciatic nerve distress. The piriformis is a muscle situated in the low buttock area on each side which attaches out of the sacrum (the triangular bone at the bottom of their spine) into the top femur, just below the hip joint.

Anatomy of this spine

A summary of the spine

The spine can be a intricate portion of one's entire body, also will be divided up to three major categories. The backbone comprises the bones which make up your backbone, such as the disks. Secondly there are neurological elements in the spinal column, like the spinal cord and nerve roots. The remaining weather of one's backbone can also be categorized as encouraging structures. These structures comprise muscles, ligaments, joints, and ligaments.

The backbone

We will center on the backbone, and this is composed of the selection of bones present on your spine, where the ribs hook up with. The spinal column serves lots of functions and purposes. When it comes to its purpose from the spine, it gives a base for attachment of both their backbone ligaments, bones, tendons, and joints. It protects the spinal cord, nerve roots, and lots of organs, and provides the major structural aid for nearly all of one's entire body, as well as the chest, shoulders, and torso. The spine gives the system proper balance and weight reduction, in addition to allows your chest to own the variety of motion it will, such as bending forwards, backward, laterally, and also rotate.

Anatomy

The spinal column is composed of both 32-34 individual nerves, which are the bones that give the cornerstone for the spinal column. These bottoms are broken up into five major categories, depending on their position on the spinal column. Starting at the bottom of the skull, then you will find seven cervical vertebrae that comprise the neck. Below those we find 12 thoracic vertebrae, found in the top rear. The decrease spine (below the curve) includes 5 nerves called cervical nerves. Located only below those, there's a set of 5 vertebrae. All these are combined, or fused with each other to generate the sacrum, that's part of the pelvis. At the lower end of this backbone is that your coccyx, or tailbone. That really is created from 3 5 fused vertebrae.

Each human vertebra is composed of several components and each has exceptional features based on the area in that it can be available. Every vertebra, no matter position, has three basic operational parts: the drum-shaped body, designed to keep weight and defy loading or compression; the anterior (back side) arch, manufactured from this lamina, pedicles and facet joints; and also, the transverse procedures, to which muscles attach.

Between every one of those pliers are intervertebral disks, usually abbreviated to only "disks". All these are constructed from quite good, hard cells which relate each vertebra into another location. They have been in the leading part of the spine and so are what provide the chest the skill to go forward, backward, laterally, and also to rotate.

Minor body injuries are a recognized fact of life for anybody who contributes a relatively busy life style. However, if pain gets debatable and chronic, it can be the time to consult with professionals concerning exactly what may possibly be the foundation of this pain. A pinched nerve can be regarded as to blame in terms of chronic pain, particularly when it develops to spine pain, neck pain, leg pain, shoulder pain or hip pain. A chiropractor might be the solution for pain relief in this circumstance, and we'll explain how to establish whether that condition may possibly be at the origin cause of one's pain.

Infection

The expression pinched nerve can be employed in medicine to explain a injury or harm to a single nerve or pair of nerves for almost any variety of explanations. The nerve mostly influenced by this affliction is that the sciatic nerve-wracking, also as it's bundles which encircle through the entire human body, it might lead to pain in are as far removed from the true injury website. As a result of the, in case you reveal the following symptoms, it could have been a smart idea to visit your regular doctor or physician instantly, so the trauma site might be ascertained, and therapy began.

Weakness: generally sensed in a extremity, such as, for instance, a leg or arm, but might usually pose itself at the back too. Is such as the muscles positioned in that field are tremendously feeble, and might lack standard strength whilst controlling them.

Tenderness: your skin, tendons and muscle inside the affected area are vulnerable to observable feelings, such as anxiety, pain, compression and extension. The complete area around the affected nerve package feels sore, such as it'd experienced acute discomfort during a very long time period.

Odd sensations: you could feel strange sensations in the affected spot, such as hooks and needles, tingling and waves of burning sensations or traumatic and changing pains. These can also coincide with muscular aches, and therefore are caused by the compression or portion of those neural bundles.

Reasons

The principal reason behind this affliction can be straightforward effort. As soon as we work hard or play hard, we run the chance of pulling muscles straining joints, and changing a number of our fragile bones out of place, particularly as we grow old. Age can be a variable for the 2nd almost certainly cause of the illness, that will be bone marrow or thickening of their bones during arthritis and aging. This may be quite a defining variable for the precise location of this compression, specially once the sciatic nerve is included.

Additional medical conditions, such as sciatica, herniated disks, and spinal stenosis could create the nerve packs across the backbone to become compacted, literally pinching the lymph vessels and also causing pain to radiate all through the human anatomy. This is the reason it's essential to be analyzed to find out the origin of the compression or injury. Too frequently the website is supposed to be at which the pain is, even if the truth is, it could be far removed as a result. Last, any injury which includes the neck, knee, spine or back may cause the vertebrae which form the spine to compress or shift, and also the spinal nerves combined with it.

Treatment options

The treatment with this illness is normally broken into stages of treatment choices. For chronic pain episodes, treatment with corticosteroid shots, accompanied by periods of bedrest, will probably alleviate the many debilitating symptoms. Chiropractic adjustments may be performed, in addition to physical therapy sessions. The trick to any workable treatment program, nevertheless, is examinations and assessments to nail the wounded location.

Can you realize that chronic pain signals traveling throughout your system quicker compared to sensory signature signs? It will and that's the reason why so many men and women use massage as an adjunct for their own pain control regimen. Ostensibly the therapists signature starts together with all the chronic pain signals traveling through the back (because this may be the pathway for several nerve-conduction) and signature wins every moment! While this could well not indicate no annoyance for you personally, it's going to absolutely mean less pain through the whole period of your massage and regularly for a time period afterward. Twist even competes with severe pain signs:(think: stub your toe) and that's the reason we instinctively reach to our hurt dig-it and hold it before the pain diminishes. Or mothers kiss a booboo. The signature signal goes faster. Regrettably the fee of massage could also be prohibitive for a great deal of individuals. 1 way to go around this would be to locate a massage school near. You may usually get an excellent massage to get a small percentage of the fee supplied by students who's over seen by an instructor. Then of course, there's always the choice of requesting a buddy or spouse to get a massage. Should you go that path you might want to get well prepared and also have some massage so that their hands will slide correctly. Nothing worse than having skin peeled from inadequate lotion or oil.

Along with while we are on the topic of chronic pain, have you noticed how stressed your muscles get when struck by an arctic burst? Our stance affects as we walk hunched over wanting to safeguard ourselves out of sub-par. If we need to stick out from sunlight for any amount of time we start to shiver, frequently with cable stressed muscles. That which can add up to is pain free in the future as we thaw out. The best remedy is prevention, so putting relaxation before fashion. I am constantly astonished at how my mature kids will groom their small ones into the hilt at the cold, however frequently wear just a fleece themselves. They laugh at me once i wear two kinds of trousers and a set of tights along with also my ill bean coat that's fantastic for 40 below after i move walking throughout subzero temperatures however, I actually don't care. I understand that layers are things keeps you warm and feel me coating such as mad! Therefore, that the next time you end up rubbing your shoulders and wondering just how they have so tender, inquire how hot you might be once you go out. The solution might surprise you.

Anatomy for fitness professionals

How to master muscular anatomy quick & prevent the 5 most shared anatomy mistakes

Anatomy = foundation of exercise science

Learning human anatomy for an exercise pro is similar to learning how to create a base being a architect; it affirms all else!

Everything else is constructed on top of it!

Personal training is very lively and romantic, therefore that i guess that you might make the exact same claim regarding personality being ; in case the client does not want to invest some time together with you as your lousy attitude or awful communication competencies, it really does not matter how far you realize!

However, that is the reason the reason why we split fitness sills in to categories. As training is indeed lively, it's effective to divide a variety of skillsets in to 3 important mega-competencies: social abilities and exercise science, and business acumen.

Anatomy and bio mechanics would be the foundation of practice science, together with physiology supplementary. (what's structure any way, except the anatomies answer to forces/mechanics? Don't hesitate to disagree from the comments, i understand that is simply not a favorite view, but i think that it really is worth analyzing)

Additionally, it doesn't matter just how far you understand about different regions of exercise science, even if you have a strong base in biomechanics and body, you won't have the capacity to safely and correctly employ your comprehension.

Different types of anatomy

Within body, you can find various targets; neural body, bony body, and muscular body. Like a trainer, it's vital to bear in mind just how a number of different structures there have been from your system which affects its operation and wellness.

Yes, initially we ought to really be centered on muscle body, however as caregivers, we must bear in mind we have a tendency to be overly dedicated to muscles some times. Many times, a tight muscle tends to tighten due to a fascial limitation! Everything is connected to all during the fascial network. Simply bear this in your mind whenever your trouble solving and analyzing.

As you progress, additional hours ought to be used learning heightened anatomy such as fascial body, and also the body of their joints, ligaments, tendons and also the way in which they connect to embryonic surfaces.

Exercise makes perfect

There is a great deal of great programs available to find body. Take advantage of these tools, the initial one is totally free, and exercise together with different coaches. Produce purchases quiz one another, and attempt to join the particular names to your exercise routine once you work out.

[anatomy for fitness] getbodysmart.com - this site is wonderful! It's an electronic digital cartoon of this muscle system. Drag on and drag just a tiny slider under each combined, and it'll construct the muscle support system round it by the deep into the superficial. Very cool and worth looking into, you may even click to observe each muscles activity, that will be good but very simplified. (make sure you browse "most frequent anatomy mistakes" below). And it's really completely free! Additionally, you will consider a quiz on the website. Every fresh fitness pro ought to know concerning this website and spending some time about it, it's good.

Person anatomy atlas of human body DVD set -this DVD collection is remarkable! I've observed all of those DVDS (the 6th one is all in regards to the organs). As soon as it's on the other side to find all 6 simultaneously, it's a excellent reference for anybody who would like to carry their own body into the second level. They ostensibly build an original cadaver facing you, together with precise animation to demonstrate each source and insertion. They begin with the rectal body, then build the muscles in deep to shallow at the top, reveal the cells from 360 viewpoints. They then reveal the neural and circulatory system, and also have connections involving each section. You might even begin with only 1 DVD at the same time, also watch only 10 minutes every day. It's fascinating! These complicated structures would be the bodies evolutionary reaction to force! DVD 1, 2, and 3 would be important for newer coaches, because they truly are upper extremity, lower extremity, and trunk/core.

Fitness anatomy strength training anatomy book - that is a superb publication. Step by step, vibrant, and just plain interesting to check at. The muscles examples have become much of a jacked human body builder, so it's maybe not exactly what you should normally find at a typical public client, however it's an awesome guide to basic human anatomy. There's perhaps not quite as much awareness to human anatomy of those "passive structures" (bones, tendons, ligaments) and spinal body.

Cadaver course - among the greatest ways to learn would be to really get your fingers dirty! I moved for the class and it was wonderful! We're so utilized to considering these cells as different, since they come in novels, however they're all merged together! This was eye opening to find the fibers of this rhomboid fan in to the fibers of this serratus! It looked just like one-muscle! Here is a URL into the site. They've a cadaver course in Pittsburgh and at Connecticut. If you're in yet another region of the earth, also you ought to have the ability to discover a cadaver class at any given university using courses that are related. The cool thing about the body optional is you're able to get continuing education credits, also it's a dependence on the resistance training professional certificate. But do not allow it to prevent you when you're not at or even Pittsburgh, look for a class and get the hands dirty!

Many common anatomiesmistake!

All these would be the largest mistakes which gym professionals and books create about body:

1. Inch. The activity of this muscular tissues is entirely determined by its own position! Yes your hip adductors move your thighs toward one another when they're abducted, but they'll expand the fashionable in the event that you're in the fashionable is fully flexed, or stretch the fashionable if it's fully flexed. If you're only beginning, aren't getting confused, simply concentrate on the obvious muscle activity, but bear in your mind that every muscles work is positional, also certainly will fluctuate dependent on the job of the joints.

2. Each muscle has some type of role in most single plane, and it's an outrageous activity, concentric activity, and isometric activity. Oh, also from every plane, " i really don't mean all of 3 airplanes since there's definitely an infinite number of airplanes (still another major yet common body mistake) what plane is cutting on out a barbell together with your own arm? In case that blows off your mind, i suggest choosing the rts certificate asap!

3. We often concentrate on shallow muscles and rectal muscles since they're easier to find and promote their dressing table! Don't make this mistake with your body or your own customers; without even equilibrium, equilibrium, and also the deeper/smaller stabilizers, you will wind up a cripple earlier or later!

4. Do perhaps not make an effort to impress your customers with your understanding of body! Naming the profound 6 trendy rotators won't impress your potential! Unless they're a physician, then they'll just be confounded and perhaps insulting! Always

confer with a client in a language that they know; that really is best for communicating and earnings. Yes, even while you create a partnership, you should enlarge your customer's knowledge in order that they simply take charge of these fitness, but then, focus going for technical comprehension and maybe not domains. At first, whenever they state "I need bigger arms, then they still seem to be older lady arms", you say"this app may specifically target people granny arms" you may sell more bundles ensured.

5. One other quick notice on speech. In all costs, avoid using the term "functional" where you ever would like simply to appear knowledgeable. Yes people want it, also it's a buzzword, however, keywords are frequently quite inefficient at communicating. Rather than "functional" state "workout or app x y z may allow you to work better in abc or function at abc or even move to activity abc". Major pet peeve of mine! Do not only sound smart when you're smart!

CHAPTER THREE

⁓

Discovering the cause of your sciatica

Infection relief for sciatica pain can be actually a must, since the pain in the bloated or injured backbone guts might be so powerful it's completely painful. The sciatic nerve is the longest nerve in the body, running in the thoracic (smallest) region of the spine from the back in to the buttocks and down the thighs. Sciatica is a disorder brought on by irritation or pressure on that nerve which travels down its length, also along with pain, it can manifest itself like being a tingling, and a weakness, or even perhaps a tingling in the affected areas.

What exactly is the spine?

The spine is a loadbearing structure comprised of twenty-five construction blocks, called vertebrae. Each vertebra is simply a couple inches wide and nearly round in look. Additionally, it features a rounded hole close to the trunk, and also the holes out of every one of the vertebrae lineups perfectly to make the backbone. Nerves from the mind operate through the backbone and then down into the rest of the entire body.

In between your vertebrae are twenty-three disks, and each roughly one quarter of a inch thick. They function as shock absorbers and cushion the bones' little movement once your human body moves. The disks, unlike the fascia, aren't composed of bone rather they truly are a material like the ribs which creates your own nose. Sciatica may be the affliction which happens once the lumbar

4 5 disk (the disk between your fifth and fourth cervical vertebrae) irritates or puts pressure on the plantar nerve developing from the backbone.

What's sciatica pain treated?

Sciatica anxiety might be treated with numerous different conventional or other modalities, like those below.

Drug

Many cases of sciatica are treated with painkillers. In very mild conditions, the primary choice is over-the-counter remedies, such as ibuprofen, acetaminophen, aspirin, or naproxen. These may help decrease the pain and commence to correct tissue at precisely the exact same moment. They're all generally regarded as safe for momentary usage of healthy adults, however you shouldn't require them for two or more weeks at one time. You also need to not have some medications containing exactly the exact same active ingredients, since you may possibly harm your liver or other organs

Exercise

Exercise is your ideal method to decrease sciatica symptoms to the very long run. By training your muscles to develop into both strong and relaxed, it's going to help cut the total amount of pressure they employ into the thoracic nerve which runs throughout them. In the event the foundation of puberty is pressure out of the short, tight piriformis muscle, the muscle has to have been softly stretched. In the event the foundation of sciatica is by the bulging disk, gentle low spine strengthening and stretching exercises can help. Yoga moves can assist with source.

workout is your reclined spinal spin. Utilize the following directions:

1. Inch. Lie flat on your back to a mat.
2. B ring up your knees to your chest, as close as possible
3. Stretch your arms to each side along with your palms down
4. Stick to the count of three.
5. Exhale into the use of five and also lower your knees slowly to the proper.
6. Sit and again bring back your knees into your own torso.
7. Exhale yet again, and also this time around lower your knees to your left side.
8. Come back into the center .
9. Repeat the exercise 8 10 times.

Earlier you start this or another workout routine, get hold of your physician or therapist to ascertain which exercises are ideal for you personally.

Alternative therapies

Fixing laughter might prove easier for several people using alternative as opposed to conventional treatments. Even though nontraditional therapies ordinarily would not need scientific proof of their advantages and security, lots of men and women find these helpful, in particular people individuals who have had no success with conventional measures.

Certainly, one of the most typical alternative remedies is chiropractic attention. Chiropractors cannot prescribe drugs, choose blood, nor do some invasive procedures, like a physician may; nevertheless, they ought to have a health history and complete physical exam, and, if justified, they could order diagnostic tests, like XRAYS and cat tests, and to decide whether there's a issue with the plantar nerve.

Chiropractors heal the full human body, together with the backbone because their specialization, and also the essence in their spinal modification therapy is dependent upon the specific reason for the sciatica. The health care provider will normally press your back to relieve swollen nerves and also boost movement on your joints. If the issue comes from a disk problem, the chiropractic way of is to alleviate anxiety to alleviate pain and restore much better motion to the spinal column joint.

Surgery

When all alternatives have failed, a physician may elect to carry out spinal operation. When herniated disks are the reason for sciatica pain, the physician may suggest doing a microdiscectomy, an operation which permanently eliminates anything is squeezing the nerve. Or, they may elect to get a discectomy, a procedure which involves removing the disk causing the issue, or the one that's laborious, in the spinal column. Once the disk was taken away, the pressure in the nerve is relieved and sciatica symptoms and pain are not reduced.

Together with treatment from sciatica, an individual has to additionally pay attention to the status which ends in the annoyance. There are lots of techniques of getting treatment from sciatica.

Sciatica causes horrendous back pain, as a result of pressure on the sciatic nerve. Sitting or standing for a protracted period or actions like biking for as long may also lead to sciatica. The damaging spreads out of the back into the buttocks and also to the foot.

To commence with, medications like aspirin, Tylenol and aspirin are normal to cut back both swelling and will also be known to decrease pain. Medicines should be obtained after a physician's management.

Second, besides medications, routine exercises may also be

invaluable in providing pain relief in sciatica. In the event there is acute pain that a couple of days of bed rest might help in relieving the discomfort but also much bedrest has a negative effect. It disturbs the muscles and as an alternative of reducing pain an individual can wind off with further pain.

Thirdly, stretching exercises and massage treatments treat muscular aches and assist in preventing pain relief from your esophagus. Muscle migraines when left untreated; often to alleviate the suffering.

Fourthly, a proper sitting position is essential to reducing the strain also to protect against an excessive amount of stress about the back. Soft mattresses or jazzy seats utilized for sitting may create worse that the illness and build a hindrance from the method of cure.

Additional compared to the people cited, averting lifting heavy objects, cold and hot compressions, several all-natural treatments for example consuming raw garlic, garlic milk, olive oil, a balanced and nutritious diet containing vitamin b 1 improved vegetables and fruits, correct intake of drinking water and a couple things that you ought to follow to treatment from sciatica.

Should you have problems with the diminished back burning pain, so it could seem as though the pain actually melts, or melts down your leg again. That is frequently connected with pain. Sometimes, individuals who have sciatica may not suffer with some true pain in their spine, but many others have problems with acute pain. For those who are afflicted with this illness that commonly causes it to feel like though your spine, leg and on occasion the medial side of one's foot is on fire, then you aren't alone, because tens of thousands of people like you have problems from this illness. Actually, it's a lot more prevalent than you may think.

Certainly, one of the best means to begin curing your spine would be to identify what's causing your pain. For a few, this could be as easy as carrying a measure erroneously and others it might possibly be something. Many men and women who suffer with burning off back pain, report which it simply happens once they go their legs into the other side, or perform tasks that want parts of these own bodies to maneuver in an unusual angle. Whenever you will find exactly what it is that creates your own spine pain to wake up, you then certainly can modify your moves in a means which won't enable one to inflame your esophagus.

Most individuals who suffer with burning lower back pain may find respite from their pain by avoiding activities that activate the debilitating reaction, but many more aren't pleased to stop performing certain things indefinitely, and those are the men and women who decided they are finished with pain drugs and being made to sit to facilitate their back pain. They will work to locate a means to permanently cure back pain.

In case this sounds just as if you then you definitely need to be aware that recent studies have unearthed your burning lower back pain could be caused by a misalignment on the human physique. To put it differently, you have any muscles which are stronger than some others. At these times, the muscles always tug each other and induce the human body to become misaligned. Which usually means that more than the poorer muscles provide up and also the stronger ones may possibly be yanking your spine to an alternative position as it should naturally function inside. For a few, the muscles are often balanced in strength till they engage in something they're not utilized to, that'll subsequently pull on the spine out of alignment and cause the burning off lower back pain that lots folks identify as sciatica.

You are able to reduce and permanently expel burning off back pain by figuring out how to offer either side of one's own body equal potency. Whether you are interested in creating a area, like the shoulders stronger and more balanced, or would like to fortify the whole spine so you are strong completely round, you're able to discover how to safely and efficiently balance your own body so you can eliminate the burning off back pain that you have problems with without pain drugs of any sort.

Just how can you know that you're having gastrointestinal nerve pain? You might feel pain on your back and also that pain will start to radiate on your buttocks and can gradually get into a own leg again. In the event you're feeling are undergoing such a pain, then you may possibly be experiencing sciatica.

Sciatica is a disorder that affects thousands of people in the whole world. From the west that it accounts for more than 80 per cent of the mature people's backpain issues. At the USA of America, over 7.5 million adults suffer with alcoholism as well as this illness is the reason its 2nd most prevalent reason people see their health practitioners each day.

The causes with the pain vary however, probably the most common of them include; a pinched sciatic nerve induced by the inflammation of the nearby joints; spinal disk herniation due to improper posture or consequent in wrongly damaging your spinal column disk whilst reaching out for something; there's yet another cause called this piriformis syndrome - that the piriformis may be that the muscle located in the buttocks; sciatica may be caused by spinal stenosis or ovarian cysts.

This informative article can look at methods by that you'll be able to find the relief you're looking for the pain. If you browse on till the conclusion, you are going to see an easy method to obtain invaluable advice relating to this illness that'll make certain you don't need to suffer out of this again on your own life. Countless people in more than 93 countries of the world used this way to treat their sciatica forever.

You are able to get relief for the own pain without even choosing for operation since a lot of individuals do. (as a primary alternative for this matter, do you think it?) Deciding on operation when you will find noninvasive operative methods to this predicament is mad. (would not you agree?)

The most common sciatic pain alleviation is choosing for maids or non-steroidal anti-inflammatory drugs. All these are all over the counter medications that help bring relief into parts of your muscles.

Subsequently there's also physical therapy including low impact exercise patterns such as; swimming, rowing, yoga, Taiichi, walking, extending and so forth. All these have the additional benefit of one's having the ability to do them in home.

Additional techniques that you may possibly like to take to are the next; massage-therapy, the usage of heat and ice packs, chiropractic methods, homeopathic treatments, the usage of blossoms and so forth.

Relieving symptoms with ice and heat

Among the ordinary confusion's folks have with self-treatment could be your matter of when to make use of ice cream and when to make use of heat. Once we discussed in the prior phase, ice hockey is more preferable once the matter is just one of nerve wracking, whilst heating is significantly better for sciatica because of muscular regeneration. In the previous chapter we discussed several hints about ascertaining the reason for one's symptoms, however if in doubt, a very simple guideline is always to base your choice of whether to use heat or ice on precisely what the signs are. When you've got intense or sharp pain without swelling, then this typically implies there was inflammation gift, also this can be a opportunity to make use of ice cream. On the flip side, if your symptoms are for the most part mild or stiffness annoyance, there's not often substantial inflammation present, also this circumstance, heat can be a much greater choice. As a precaution, unless you've undergone a trauma, or think it's likely you have injured yourself, it's ideal to refrain from heat for at least 4-8 hours to be certain the inflammatory response will not be triggered and the redness has not had enough time to install. When in doubt, stay clear of heat! Even though heat might feel well although it's on (because heat increases transmission of certain neural signals which hurt signs to be somewhat obstructed by achieving the brain), heat increases the inflammatory response to the human anatomy. Increased inflammation means raised pain whenever you quit using heat. Even though ice might well not seem too comfortable as heating, it really is among the very best anti-inflammatory measures you may take. The temporary disquiet of employing ice usually pays in long-term aid. Even though some experts recommend alternating heat and ice (as an instance, 10 minutes of ice hockey accompanied by 10 minutes of heat), i haven't seen any specific advantage by this way. In most cases, choosing one or another predicated on the outward symptoms as was only discussed is usually the easiest way and within my own experience works only as well or better than wanting to substitute the remedies. No matter whether you're employing heat or ice, you always need to divide the hot or ice bunch out of skin using a coating of fabric to reduce skin damage. It's likewise essential to avoid using heat or ice on a place that's been treated with, icy hot, bio freeze, ben-gay, or even any further topical ointment - wait before impression of this analgesic has worn away, otherwise the heat or ice can lead to skin damage or annoyance.

Additionally, when utilizing either heat or ice, you should only use the procedure for approximately 1-5 minutes at one time, allowing your skin to return to normalcy temperature (to be safe and allow 1 or 2 hours) prior to applying the treatment. Because it could have a couple of minutes to your cold or hot sensation to produce it through the cloth layer between your cold/hot pack as well as skin, start time when you begin to feel that the temperature shift on the epidermis area.

Crucial note*: if you've got diminished flow or diminished skin sensitivity because of nerve injury, diabetes, etc., and it's ideal to consult with your health care provider first before employing heat or ice.

Sciatica symptom relief exercises

There are various exercises which were indicated for its self-treatment of sciatica. I frequently encounter individuals who've been awarded long, complicated lists of exercises by either doctors or physical therapists. The majority of those exercises are of nominal benefit in the optimal and on account of the intricacy of the physical exercise regime, many patients do not utilize them to get long-term. In my 20 plus years of clinical experience have discovered that using a few especially effective exercises to an average basis is a lot more beneficial than just having patients perform a whole lot of unique exercises. Within this phase, i will be introducing exercise tips which are designed to relieve pain as fast as achievable. While major ailments are found, i recommend that an "intensive care" way into the exercises at which frequent reproduction is the trick to symptom relief. The idea of copying is just one which i do wish to highlight because I've given these tips to tens of thousands of people through the past few years throughout my chiropractic office in addition to my blogs and online instructional videos and also the requirement for frequent reproduction in early phases of treatment is always missed. That is probably simply because of the manner that exercises are normally exhibited by health practitioners and physicians. The typical manner that exercises for sciatica have been exhibited is the affected individual has been led by them at a physician's or therapist's office at a supervised treatment session lasting 15 to 30 minutes together with treatment sessions daily or another day, or so the patient is only supplied a sheet of exercises and also told to complete them in your home. In the beginning, together with all these procedures, the patient does the exercises one or two times every day. For neural compression sciatica linked to a bulging disc, which is inadequate to acquire lasting relief speedily, therefore patients may frequently select all weeks or months in pain using very slow advancement.

Today you might be convinced that is clearly a lot - and it's also, but the majority of individuals won't need to maintain up this frequency for long. Typically, a couple days into a couple weeks of multiple times a hour utilization of those exercises i am going to show will radically lower the symptoms, so when this does occur, you're able to decrease the frequency of these exercises into merely several minutes daily to avoidance (as we'll discuss in the chapter about prevention and rehab). The particular frequency of these exercises may vary significantly in line with this individual. As a rule of thumb, for individuals up to approximately 50 decades old, it is suggested starting with doing each exercise for about one minute at one time in a frequency of 5 to 6 days daily. For folks over 50, i would recommend you start with a frequency of roughly 50% that at two to three times each day. That is only because elderly individuals frequently have a certain amount of arthritis, which is temporarily annoyed by the indicated exercises. Lots of men and women would find some good discomfort inside their shoulders or backs throughout the "intensive maintenance" period of their exercises. That may be temporary, and may typically be eased with using ice as discussed earlier in the day, and/or using massage. Provided that the soreness is still tolerable, i suggest continuing with all the exercises at the recommended frequency, however you always have the option to lessen the frequency of this exercise if needed. 1 final point of clarification before i move in to the exercises will be that the simple fact from the perspective of the overall health of nerves, numbness is much worse than annoyance. Even though the majority of men and women notice numbness to become comfortable compared to pain, tingling indicates longer or greater interval nerve compression compared to pain really does. Consequently, if you're beginning mostly together with numbness also it really is shifting to pain, then that's in fact a fantastic sign ordinarily. On the flip side, should you begin with mostly pain and it's shifting to numbness, that's often a poor sign and is still an indicator you need to change what you're doing or find professional therapy. That said it's crucial to tell apart numbness, and it is a deficiency of sense, from "heaviness" or"fatigue" that sometimes does occur for a brief period after acute pain goes off. If you are uncertain that you're having, gently jab the effected area having a needle or pin (that you really don't have to break skin) and compare the impression to the very same area across the other side of one's own body or yet another area that feels ordinary and also compare them. In case the pin/needle feels roughly the exact same on either areas, you're most likely simply experiencing heaviness leading to muscles relaxing since the neural soreness diminishes.

Mckenzie procedure (called for physical therapist robin McKenzie) are frequently related to expansion (backward bending) of their spine, in reality they're about analyzing, after which exercising, stretches and positions which facilitate or produce "centralization" of outward symptoms. Centralization signifies that the outward symptoms proceed nearer into the spinal column. As an instance, when you've got low back pain with sciatica (leg pain), then centralization are at which in fact the observable symptoms leave or decrease at the leg, then even when pain remains the exact same or gets worse at the buttocks or even low back again.

Perhaps you are aware about prostate massage and you're wondering why "how i could utilize prostate massage that will help my climax?" well, this sensual massage may truly be a enormous assistance give your guy a trackable discharge. However, "just how would you do precisely that?" I've got the solution for both questions.

You can utilize the prostate massage as a way to present your man an alternative sort of orgasm. It's a discharge that could be tremendously intense when compared with the customary orgasm he's. Some men that have tried this strategy assert this is the man variation of multiple climaxes. If done correctly with caution, the bliss will absolutely follow along with

If you're prepared to assist your person attain prostate orgasm, then you must prepare yourself with the odd procedure of researching the interiors of the anus. Don't stress. There's a suitable means that you safely perform so massage. You don't need to feel afraid that you may damage your individual. Provided that you follow my hints, you are just going to be fine.

First thing you need to accomplish is to speak to your partner with regards to your sake of wanting this particular massage. You can not only surprise him as this may possibly hamper the catastrophic effect of this experience. It took me my fan sometime until we successfully reached vaginal climax. It needs a considerable quantity of time and a great deal of patience.

Some of the first problems you need to manage will be the positioning. You will kneel before your partner while he's standing. Take your hands between his thighs, and hit out because of his butt with your hands before you personally. When he fails to feel more comfortable with this particular position, you might just ask him to lie on his back and then open his or her legs. Within this position you can easily get his prostate and penis.

You're absolutely free to detect different places that could do the job with you both. I recommend you don't rush to converse in your own very first effort. Only go slow. Start with being comfortable with only touching his ass. You will touch his manhood as you're researching his anal area. This will be quite gratifying for him personally.

It's not exactly about the massage and also the processes. It's also wise to let your fan believe that you're appreciating the sight, so that you like what you're doing. This are the ideal turnon for the partner. When he sees that you also receive pleasure from pleasing himhe would be happy. Thus, make eye contact and speak with him as you're carrying out these.

All these are the necessities that you might want once you try so prostate massage: caliber paper and paper towels. The lubricant will assist you along with your partner using penetration. You really do want decent lubricant at there because his anal area isn't utilized for the sort of sensation. To help relieve his muscles and also to produce the penetration smooth, then the lubricant may help you.

Paper towels are for the litter you may possibly create. With the typical orgasm, the consequences of this discharge is a lot thinner. Inside this massage, the semen will be watery and also the total amount will be greater. That is a result of the fluid out of his prostate. Thus, prepare yourself with a paper towels which means that you might prevent the mess.

Proceed and research with your own man. I promise you he is going to be pleased with the prostate massage you'll likely be providing him. At this time, you're already targeted with the suitable knowledge that'll permit one to employ prostate massage that will assist you to man orgasm.

Even as we grow old are muscles and tendons become stiffer. For lots of individuals their own bodies also have undergone multiple cycles of trauma, inflammation and pain, some level of reimbursement in the region of trauma, and version of their surrounding tissues, ligaments and tendons. Once the redness subsides as well as the pain has been eliminated, either from medications or rest, they believe that they have been treated. Regrettably, these injuries frequently lead to misaligned joints which don't go as well and muscular adhesions causing decreased endurance. Your system will adaptively go on to prevent pain throughout this episode. Based upon the length of pain and the quantity of structures required a specific level of reimbursement does occur. All this results on your own body changing how it moves and conveys it self.

In otherworld's movement routines vary now follow the course of least resistance. With the years the quantity of muscle fibers ready for movement gets lessoned. Other organs are used wrongly and eventually become shortened or lengthened. This leads to pain and weakness in many regions of the human anatomy. Your human anatomy farther adjusts or compensates by changing our posture to accommodate to the fluctuations in joints and muscles. Additionally, the limitation in joint movement places additional pressure on the ligaments, muscles and fibrocartilage leading to degenerative joint modifications. The associated joint limitation additionally leads to changed messages being sent and received throughout the nervous system, leading to further aberrations of function and movement. The consequent cycle leads to complex aging of localized muscle and joint tissues. The consequent cycle frequently suppresses easy motion and movement. Statistically, the inability to perform is connected to earlier mortality.

Besides adjustments of movement, our stance, how we balance your human body will be also interrupted. Altered neurological signs from joint dysfunction or restriction allow it to be harder to balance. Research shows that elderly individuals with inadequate balance possess a increased prevalence of drops. What's more, research in the older states that decreasing can be a elevated risk for sooner mortality. Additionally, forward head posture contributes to higher chance of drops. Rounding of their shoulders and also tightening of their anterior torso muscles lead to diminished capacity to breath and could donate to cardio pulmonary issues.

Now it's simple to learn how poor posture, motion and balance might bring about complex aging and sooner departure, however do posture and chiropractic exercise effect that this procedure. Chiropractic works by finding and repairing joints which can be mis aligned and secured. Adjustments restore normal posture and motion inside the combined rendering it less difficult to go. Additionally, the alteration leads to the routine transmission of neural signals from the brain into your human body as well as human body. This ordinary nerve wracking is vital for appropriate balance and muscular contraction, in addition to for the organs to operate correctly. Restoring suitable position into the combined with all the alteration allows for superior alignment of body cells. Chiropractic frequently incorporates acupuncture techniques into regions of muscles leading to the breaking up of adhesions and enhanced motion and endurance. Once the joints have been unlocked and emptied in the alterations, and also the muscles relaxed and stretched by the massage methods, your own body is prepared to be re trained to proceed and hold it self. The effective use of particular postural rehab exercises helps retrain muscles to maneuver correctly and balance exercises help individuals hold our own body at an even far more aligned posture. The mixture of chiropractic adjustments, stretching and massage processes and also exercises that are concentrated permit favorable changes within our balance, movement and recovery. These positive impacts permit us to proceed better even as we age and better accommodate to the outside pressures your system confronts a daily basis. In conclusion, the favorable affects inside the own body as a consequence of the use of posture and chiropractic exercises create a change of these conditions described previously that contribute to premature mortality and aging. As a result of the, posture and chiropractic exercises may be referred to as an anti-fungal therapy.

CHAPTER FOUR

❧

Natural remedies sciatica

Sciatica is an enormous problem on earth these days. Even though there are lots of diverse treatments for a natural cure for sciatica pain appears to become the ideal. Lots of people seek out an all purely natural remedy but few actually gain in the so called all-natural cure for pain. It's crucial that you learn that sciatica itself just isn't actually a disease, but a disorder triggered by a pair of different illnesses such as a bulging or herniated disk, spinal stenosis, spondylolisthesis, injury, piriformis syndrome, and spinal nerves.

Natural remedy for sciatica

Here we've got some all-natural treatments which could help relieve you of your sciatica pain when properly used along with daily physical exercise.

*juices from berries and celery leaves will provide relief if drunk at minimum number of 10 oz daily. If you put in beet roots and carrots for the mix it is going to get an improved taste and it may also intensify the consequence with the natural remedy.

Decision elderberry tea is really a called muscle relaxant and stimulant and may cure sciatica indications.

*you may also choose garlic nutritional supplements to assist with the pain. In the event you decide to simply take garlic supplements i would advise that you never require a lot more than is reportedly studied on the tag. Consuming raw garlic or taking garlic supplements together with other supplements of vitamin b 1 and complex gives relief from pains and aches, helps flow, is definitely an anti-oxidant and provides your body with warmth and also energy. A great treatment for sciatica is garlic . Only grab two tsp of garlic and then sit in a cup of milk and then beverage this two per day and you'll see results so on.

*another bewitching home remedy to deal with sciatica is brand new minced horseradish poultice, that when put on the painful places and retained for an hour or so at one period arouses the thoracic nerve and also provides immense relief from stomach pain.

A natural treatment for sciatica pain might be quite beneficial but remember to include things like a fantastic eating plan, regular training and also you have to remember that you're intending to boost your general wellbeing. If you would like to avoid with this issue occur again later on you might choose to sleep on a firm mattress. Consistently sit stand in good position, and also stay away from lifting heavy items just as far as feasible. It's the smaller things which cause sciatica pain at the very long haul, therefore make sure you make this part of one's daily routine. Many could find it challenging to stick to those organic patterns.

Sciatica is amongst the common ailments affecting lots of people throughout their life. As stated by the national institutes of health at the USA, it's the 2nd most frequent neurological disorder reported. Only annoyance surpasses it at frequency of reported cases. Its origin is more varied; it may be as naive as a very simple muscle injury or trauma to complicated problems like disk problems, spinal stenosis, osteoporosis, or even cancerous tumors. Oftentimes acupuncture to get sciatica pain alleviation and other organic remedies are all that's required to relieve the pain with the frequent condition.

In case you have spine pain it's sensible to pay for a trip to a own family physician because only your physician can exclude the serious reasons for your back pain. In addition, when addressed and fulfilled head, there's not any sort of sciatica that may not be readily attacked therefore you can find rest from pain.

If, as is likely your pain is the result of a strain or trauma to a lower spine, treatments available are both straightforward and numerous. You also might opt to approach your anxiety in a conventional way, together with exercises to strengthen your heart muscles and treatment drugs or, as the majority are currently doing, process your therapy at a more holistic manner, natural method. On the list of holistic methods accessible are acupuncture, acupuncture, herbal medicine, and noninvasive all-natural methods.

The range of natural remedies, particularly such as trauma or anxiety, offer powerful treatment together with not one of the unwanted shared with medication therapy. Natural methods for treatment tend to be more affordable and more conservative compared to conventional medical procedures to this issue of spine pain. Accepting maids for pain within long spans, as an instance, a conventional strategy, may render you with liver disease, bleeding sores and might even result in death from complications of those unwanted side effects. Some medications relieve pain from dulling pain receptors within your mind. A client of mine that had been on Ultram for pain once clarified the pills because "dumb pills" due to how that it made him feel.

Natural treatments for spine pain

Acupuncture: traditional Chinese medicine including acupuncture because a simple treatment option is dependent on the thought that the chi or life force may get obstructed, which the stations which disperse chi during the human body is able to be discharged through the appropriate insertion of thin needles at the complete points which restrain the chi for the individual complaint. Oftentimes, acupuncture together with a simple program of practice is sufficient to bring back one to pain free residing in a couple weeks.

Eazol: lots of folks swear with this particular natural, cosmetic item. Made of botanical ingredients such as willow bark, lobelia and Boswellia, eazol behaves to lubricate your muscles and also relieve stress in muscular. Additionally, it functions like a safe method to relieve pain.

Yoga: the Indian app of posture meditation and control is a type of exercise which, when directed by a specialist may help relieve the pain of back pain. That isn't any age or sex restriction on the tradition of yoga.

Sexy baths: though ice is ideal for reducing redness, warmth functions to flake out bloated muscle tissues and also behave as a direct supply of relief for the pain. Insert movement like this of a whirlpool and put in sexy tub oils like peppermint or lavender and also the pain-relieving nature of the petroleum adds to this experience. Lots of men and women who take to this adventure hours of aid. Included with some routine of exercise, hot tubs are a really real supply of relief.

Antioxidants and minerals: there are a number of vitamins which are regarded as quite effective for back treatment including vitamin b 12, vitamin, vitamin d, vitamin chamomile along with also others.

Thus there you own it. Natural methods to treatment are a true choice. Acupuncture for sciatica treatment is a high selection but other organic choices may also be offered. Because every situation is different you will need to find which ones work with you.

Obviously, remember to always bring exercise for the heart.

People frequently refer shortness pain for a type of disorder, yet this idea is definitely false as this annoyance refers to an undeniable simple fact which you're likely experiencing the herniated disk and also the pain is its own only symptom. Therefore what's the natural treatment for sciatica pain which might be imbibed on your own life to realize some type of relief? Stretches are usually recommended in addition to the ingestion of drugs, but some times is preferred, to assess with a physician or physiotherapist to become certain the exercises have been done precisely.

Celery leaves juices or juices containing potatoes can relieve the pain whenever they're consumed at the number often oz on a normal basis. For those that are already swallowing anti-coagulation drugs or suffering from illnesses like nausea, should choose prior advice from their physician before swallowing the garlic established supplements. If those juices don't agree with your taste buds, and then it is possible to alter your attention to carrot established tea, since it's well known to possess similar sort of ramifications.

Routine ingestion of garlic supplements can't just offer you plenty of energy but in addition, it serves as a superb type of pure cure for pain. Rather than popping vitamin b1 supplements, you also may add foodstuffs such as bread, poultry, legumes, green beans on what you eat in order it helps boost up the degree of vitamin b1 from your system which then can lessen the degree of the sciatica pain.

Sexy and cold packs may perhaps work as wonders because an all-natural cure for pain. Throughout the very first stages of their annoyance, cold packs might also be placed on the affected area for a period of time of roughly twenty-five minutes, often times daily. After a period of a couple of days, you may initiate the using packs and then onwards may utilize both the kinds of packs rather to relieve pain. These packs may enhance the degree of blood flow within your system and consequently it's a successful tool to lower the high level of the stomach pain. With the amalgamation of those herbal treatments it is easy to deal up with the back pain.

Hip anxiety can be quite debatable as it could confine the movement of their human anatomy, treatments may offer relief and also promote smooth and hassle free moves. There are lots of causes of hip pain, so the thigh-bone called femur swivels from the socket in cool to combine top and lower chest of your system and offer joint movement. There's some free space from the socket that gets full of fluid and blood if there's any swelling or disease at the joint. Other structures connected with the joint may be the foundation of annoyance. In the majority of the cases injury is the principal reason for pain. Though stylish pain might be debatable but sometimes referral pain can be also experienced in trendy such as the main one in the instance of irritated thoracic nerve. Arthritis also can trigger hip pain, muscular strain or strained joints can also be commonly found grounds of hip painkillers.

Perhaps not straining the aching section of this trendy throughout the flow while sitting, getting out of bed or bending is just a preventative step to prevent annoyance of this pain. The pain may possibly have been caused because of strained muscle or tendon that may become additional girth if pressure has been exerted onto it throughout any given activity. It may appear that cold and hot compresses would be unable to help as pain is deep inside however it isn't correct, cold and hot compresses could be exceedingly good all-natural cure for hip pain although compressions will likely be implemented for longer duration compared to pain at different regions of the human body. Soft massage in the painful area can be also helpful, pain relieving lotions or gels are also useful for massagetherapy. The massage will likely be achieved with adequate pressure too much nor too much. Massage boosts the flow of blood and therapies swelling and alleviates strained muscles to relieve the pain.

Care may be obtained while sitting and waking out of bed so that an excessive amount of pressure isn't handed down into the bothering location. While sitting softly folding and unfolding straight leg helps if pain is a result of slight overtraining. Leisurely walk wearing horizontal soul shoes is likewise beneficial in boosting the flow of blood and treating discomforts from the fashionable.

Capsaicin ointment can be obtained as over the counter medicine on the current market and can be an exceptional all-natural pain-relieving lotion. This lotion is composed of pepper that decelerates the signs of pain becoming moved to brain. Ergo a individual feels diminished pain and no pain as a result of its own application. Though this isn't a remedy but respite from pain may aid for making movement and enhancing relaxation.

In case a individual feels shooting pain that's radiating down to thighs compared to this lotion could be helpful because a result a nuisance may result from aggravation of thoracic nerve. Adding the entire body below midsection in bathtub full of heated water and 2 cups of Epsom salt can be a powerful all-natural remedy to relieve hip pain when caused because of muscle cramps or strains. Epsom salt includes calcium that's when consumed by the human body via skin alleviates this type of annoyance. Eating fruits and vegetable, greater ingestion of garlic from your diet, with ginger in foods like in salad along with avoiding red meat and hot food additionally works nearly as good cure for hip pain.

In case you're handling sciatica then you almost certainly understand the pain that's related to that. Handling pain on your back, legs and sometimes even your buttocks could make it rather tricky to work in life. Doing the tiniest tasks might be exceedingly complicated and debilitating. For this reason, you might choose to come across some remedies for sciatica which will work and allow you to relieve the pain.

Naturally, there will be several medications which might succeed when it has to do with decreasing the pain which you will well be experiencing. Some healthcare experts will prescribe anti-inflammatory drugs. The others might enhance muscle relaxants. A lot of people have even found rest out of over-the-counter drugs. You may always should talk with your physician in order they will have the ability to ascertain what kind of medication is going to soon be the right for you personally.

Once the pain has begun to diminish, and you're finding some relief, so you might well be invited to go to physical therapy. You may obtain this to be somewhat useful as the therapist will be in a position to provide you a few programs and exercises which could possibly find a way to help reduce the chance of harms later on. Participants are also educated on what best to improve position and maximize their flexibility in order they don't become injured.

In very acute scenarios, once you aren't getting relief from every other sorts of treatments, your physician might recommend surgery. This program will frequently simply be indicated if you're experiencing fatigue, your intestines are affected with the strain on the guts or your own pain is ongoing to make worse.

Of course, there will be several remedies which you can employ in your home to attempt to diminish the pain which you're having. It might be an advantage to one personally to put a cold pack on the debilitating for about 20 minutes every day. Next, you might find relief should you attempt to substitute cold and heat packs every afternoon. Just ensure you are using your heating pack on the bottom setting.

People who are searching for alternative therapy techniques might decide to try chiropractic services or perhaps acupuncture. It's important to not forget that not all individuals will discover respite from these types of options. Consequently, it's going to be crucial that you take to unique things to find out what's going to help you . You can even talk with your physician prior to hand to see what they can urge.

Natural anti-inflammatories

Pain, swelling, stiffness.. All these are simply a couple words that people use when describing their osteoarthritis. Medicines such as ibuprofen and aspirin can provide quick relief, however they could also result in unwanted side effects when used within a protracted time period. Many vitamin supplements and herbs, by comparison, can provide long-term safe treatment of these pains and pains associated with osteoarthritis. When thinking of a specific nutritional supplement or herb, tips are centered on how much research can be found to encourage its own effectiveness.

Many research studies indicate that glucosamine sulfate supplements can be useful in relieving the symptoms of arthritis. They do so by increasing a jelly-like compound called mucopolysaccharides to boost the shock-absorbing land of joints and inhibiting the elastase receptor, that results in the damage of joints. Studies have also suggested that supplements containing chondroitin sulfate could be helpful; those work by arousing lactic acid, which subsequently increases viscosity from the combined space. If agent turns out to become effective, still another viable choice could be that the nutritional supplement same (s-adenyl methionine). Like glucosamine, sam e is a compound that prevents corrosion of the joint.

Certain herbs may be helpful in the cure of gout. The anti-inflammatory element of devil's claw might offer relief, along with a infusion of avocado/soybean oils was demonstrated to decrease stiffness and pain related to arthritis. Phytodolor is a anti-inflammatory herb mixture made up of ash, aspen and golden rod that could reduce symptoms also. Studies have also demonstrated that niacinamide, a sort of b vitamin based from niacin, might work in relieving pain and swelling. To get a simple and reasonably priced alternative, consider drinking a cup of sour cherry juice each day. Tart cherries are demonstrated to have an potent anti-inflammatory effect, that may be specially valuable in relieving mild cases of arthritis.

Before you go into the retail store, be sure to did your research regarding the services and products that you may be thinking about purchasing. There are tools available offering evaluations and information regarding various herbs and supplements. Bear in your mind to start looking for supplements and never this is the most economical choice; perhaps not all supplements are created equally, and also the most economical supplements aren't always the ideal alternative.

Also remember that seeking the proper treatment solution is dependent upon a individual's individual preferences, demands, along with also condition. Therefore, it is very critical that you consult to your physician before choosing a nutritional supplement or supplement. To initiate the dialog you might state,"i'm interested in choosing supplements. What would you imagine?" this promotes an open conversation and promotes a more collaborative experience along with your medical care provider as a way to ascertain the most effective policy for you.

In present day medicine you will find numerous diverse things which can be utilised to help with treatment for men and women that have chronic reoccurring issues, including lots of all-natural supplements. Certainly one of the most recent improvements to the lineup, maxgxl, supports your entire body's production of glutathione, a enormous anti-inflammatory agent which may definitely offer you a great deal of assistance people who find they're afflicted by issues like rheumatoid arthritis and allergies, which may result in problems when coping with swelling and swelling. This effective anti-oxidant can offer treatment for individuals that have been required to take care of chronic problems for many, many years.

The simple fact that glutathione can be really a enormous anti-inflammatory is another incentive for the many terrific properties. Initially, little was understood about it pure chemical aside from the simple fact it worked wonders being a antioxidant which helped cleanse your body of toxins which was deposited into our systems on a normal basis. But various studies have proven it is often associated with many different crucial roles in the system, pain alleviation being merely one of them. Additionally, it has been discovered that low amounts of atherosclerosis can lead to a individual to degenerate quicker, as their bodies are unable to neutralize the components which accelerate up era factors such as toxins and free radicals.

Because it's been unearthed that treatment can be inserted into this listing of glutathione advantages also, that really is really something of a blessing into the organic medicine armory, especially considering, too, which glutathione is really a enormous anti-aging agent. Once we get older, the creation of pure glutathione in your system reduces therefore to be able to be certain all organs and organs are working in their greatest degrees, it is crucial that you take antidepressant supplements. In reality, lots of have already chose to bring this supplement to their own everyday vitamin regimen to be certain they receive the potent outcomes with the amino acid chemical. Maxgxl is this kind of supplement which supports collagen manufacturing.. And it's natural and organic.

There are certainly a couple common deficiencies which could cause tenderness and sciatica-like pain. A scarcity of all the b vitamins could possibly activate various nerve-related symptoms such as shortness. Of each the b vitamins, lack might be most common in b 6 and b 12. With respect to vitamin b 6 lack, the lack can be due to a lowered ability of your system to convert the vitamin into the active form called pyridoxal-5-phosphate (also called p5p), instead of a deficiency of ingestion of b6. Because of this i suggest having a supplement which comprises at least portion of this b6 from the pyridoxal-5-phosphate sort. From a dose perspective, i would suggest supplementing using 30 to 50 milligrams of pyridoxal-5-phosphate every day. Much like vitamin b 6 lack, vitamin b12 lack is frequently brought more to factors aside from daily ingestion. Vitamin b 12 asks a chemical created by the human body referred to as "intrinsic factor" to be consumed and utilized. Production of inherent variable will frequently be decreased in elderly individuals and those who have a history of alcohol misuse. Because diminished inherent variable prevents the absorption of vitamin b- 12, although supplementation using high oral doses of b 12 in solid shape might well not be enough to fix the lack of in these scenarios, scarcity can be adjusted with periodic shots of liquid vitamin b 12 by a certified health provider, or sub-lingual supplementation. Sub lingual liquid vitamin b12 isn't as easily obtainable as powerful supplements and isn't designed to be consumed, but stored from the mouth under the tongue to get absorption straight into the blood flow during the mucous membranes of your mouth area. Before proceeding using b-12 injections or sub-lingual supplementation, then it's strongly advised that the blood testing has been done in order to ascertain whether there is really a vitamin b12 deficiency. Dosing is dependent upon the concentration of this nutritional supplement used along with the area of the lack of yet another frequent lack that could create sciatica-like outward symptoms is nutrient lack. Fat deficiency is most frequently found in those who lose plenty of fluid during sweat, nausea, vomiting, or nausea, as well as in people with kidney disorder. Additionally, it may occur as a side effect of certain medications, like those for hypertension - notably diuretics. Mild potassium deficiency can typically be adjusted safely simply by gaining more potassium from diet. Even though peanuts would be the traditional high-potassium food, a number of different foods really are of the same quality or even better sources of potassium. These generally include melons, oranges, avocados, many green leafy veggies, and black-strap molasses. Vitamin supplements will also be available, however before taking high doses of vitamins nutritional supplements, it's strongly suggested that blood testing has been performed to quantify cholesterol levels - an excessive amount of potassium may be dangerous! 1 other lack that could make sciatica-like outward symptoms, but usually as part of all-over human body pain, would be co-enzyme q 10 (or even coq-10 for short). This lack is frequently the consequence of a disadvantage of esophageal drugs. There are just two options in tackling the lack. The foremost will be to supplement with coenzyme q 10 at an recommended starting dose of 200 milligrams every day. If it relieves symptoms, then the dose can normally be reduced to 50 to 100 milligrams every day for maintenance. When there isn't any benefit, and symptoms usually do appear to be associated with cholesterol lowering drugs, it's advisable that this issue be discussed with your doctor as well as maybe you are able to switch to an alternative medication or talk alternatives to permit one to log off of this drug altogether. Even though co-enzyme q 10 is generally secure and well-tolerated, it can have the capacity to narrow the bloodstream, and thus if you're on aspirin therapy or even more powerful anabolic medication (for example, coumadin), then you should speak to your health care provider or pharmacist prior to starting pancreatic q 10. In the end, even though perhaps not technically a lack, some diabetics may experience symptoms from the legs which may be confused for sciatica which can be linked to nerve damage resulting from diminished flow. These indicators will often be helped by supplementation with alpha lipoic acid, and it is just a strong anti-inflammatory. For long-term usage, a regular dose of roughly 50 milligrams each day is suggested. Bigger doses are occasionally suggested for short-term usage, but should just be performed under the oversight of a healthcare professional.

Prevention of sciatica

Should you have a pain which awakens out of down your back to a buttock and leg, and then you probably have sciatica. This excruciating pain is due from the most rapid guts of your system termed the sciatic nerve which runs from the back into a buttock and cool and down back of the thighs. It's generally a symptom of some other disease and the length of time it can take for that pain to disappear completely is based upon the reason.

Which exactly are the signs of sciatica? Here are the typical symptoms of the illness:

- you suffer from pain which could differ from a mild annoyance to exceptionally embarrassing. It radiates from the back into a buttock and down the back of the calf and thigh.
- your muscles feel helpless and there can be tingling.
- you get a tingling sensation plus even a pin-and-needles sensation,

frequently from the feet.

- symptoms have been aggravated because of prolonged sitting and coughing or coughing.
- there may possibly become described as a lack of bowel or bladder control which requires emergency maintenance.

Which exactly are the causes?

As mentioned previously, this illness requires the sciatic nerve which controls lots of muscles of the calves. If something compresses the origin cause of the nerve located inside the lower back, you go through the signs of sciatica. A herniated disk in the lower spine may be the most frequent reason behind the compression. Disks are made of cartilage and also are observed between the vertebrae in your spine. They act as shock absorbers whenever you proceed. With age, these discs start to deteriorate resulting from the jellylike substance during this disc to float from their outer covering of this disc drive. That is known as disc or herniation. Whilst the herniated disc presses on a nerve root, this causes pain in your leg or back.

Lumbar spinal stenosis, spondylolisthesis, piriformis syndrome, and adrenal glands are a few of the different illnesses which might result in sciatica.

Age, excessive bending of the spine, taking heavy loads, forcing for lengthy periods, prolonged sitting, and diabetes are a few of the things which put you at a risk with this particular illness.

What's sciatica diagnosed?

Together with rest and time, the illness usually gets improved. But when the pain persists for over one month or becoming progressively more demanding, medical assistance is necessary. Your doctor will conduct an entire physical exam, specially of one's spine and thighs. Some primary tests like walking in your feet or heels will probably be utilised to look at on your muscular strength and girth.

The doctor can suggest an imaging test like a spinal xray, mri, or ct scan when the pain is more intense to eliminate other causes.

The best way to treat sciatica?

Self-care measures like cold or hot packs, overthecounter medications, and extending work well in relieving the symptoms of sciatica. For those who have a herniated disc, then your personal doctor might recommend physical therapy accompanied by rehabilitation therapy once the pain improves. Laughter treatment will contain exercises to strengthen your muscles, and improve your endurance, and adjust your own posture. It's going to assist in preventing recurrent accidents. Prescribed medications like anti-inflammatory medications and muscle relaxants for reducing the redness and relieving the irritation might also be guided by your personal doctor.

Steroidal injections or surgeries like microdiscectomy could possibly be indicated if conservative measures don't alleviate the annoyance.

There are those who've profited by using other remedies like acupuncture, massage, chiropractic, and acupuncture too.

Sciatica therapy exercises can't just maintain your spine healthy later on, but might work to get back pain at this time in the event that you realize the proper ones and also how to complete them. In the event you suffer with sciatica, then you're no stranger to this pain this illness might cause. Maybe you simply take control the counter or prescription pain relievers, however you have to be aware there is yet another, more natural means to alleviate the pain and also protect against upcoming sciatica pain permanently. Many caregivers advise that you start exercising instantly, since this really is the very best approach to find the treatment you require. Thus, escape bed and start curing your spine and relieving your back pain.

Sciatica anxiety is due when the nerves have been rubbed or compacted. This may lead to an unpleasant burning sensation that runs down the leg into the foot and frequently the pain may become so acute it could be hard to go. This is exactly the reason why nausea exercises are therefore essential, because they function to fortify either side of the spine muscles and also prevent pulling of their spine in any one direction. This assist keep the spine correctly coordinated and protect against prospective stress on the sciatic nerve.

Not just in the event you're doing sciatica training exercises to avoid your pain today, however it is necessary to adopt an everyday workout routine that targets keeping the heart and spine muscles strong and that means it's possible to prevent future troubles with your digestive tract wracking. In the event you are afflicted with disk troubles, then you will likely even discover that a fantastic solid exercise routine could continue to keep them healthy as well and this may prevent problems like slipped and herniated discs.

Just what exactly sciatica therapy exercises if you be doing today?

Exercises which will fortify your'heart' with muscle relaxation therapy, however, can train your muscles to take part as a way to assist one to remain healthy and powerful. They're a terrific method to be certain the spine and heart are both robust and equipped to interact to maintain your body moving without injury to either disks or the plantar nerve.

Now you also need to think of sciatica exercises which enable one to extend your spine muscles. Since the spine muscles may grow at different speeds and one negative can be stronger, it generates tenseness from the trunk. As time passes, these stressed muscles will tug in the backbone and may create stress on the stomach muscles. By doing sciatica exercises, then you also are able to keep your muscles prevent yanking both sides, and this could continue to keep your spine straight and impartial.

When done each day, such as contraceptive treatment exercises can enable one to own a powerful, pain-free back and core to lifetime, regardless of what you end up doing.

CHAPTER FIVE

❦

The solution to prevention and recovery

With the exclusion of these few cases whenever there is structural damage to the true spine due to bulging disks or spinal stenosis, exercises for sciatica treatment would be just the ticket that you require for a comprehensive recovery. In the rare instances of structural triggers of the low backpain, strengthening the heart muscles might assist you to avert or, at the lowest, delay more revolutionary operation.

The center muscle tissue which encourage that the backbone are usually one of the most neglected muscle groups from your system yet these muscles, even should cared of regularly, offer you the best prevention against toenails readily available. What's more astonishing is the fact that the exercises demanded can be achieved before you get out of bed each daytime. Ten minutes each day and you also decrease the danger of back pain significantly.

Next-to chronic headache, back pain and tenderness pain has become really the most familiar of most neurological disorders based on the national institutes of health. As it's very prevalent, lots of men and women wonder why there's not any fantastic means to safeguard against the distress and pain due to inflammation of the sciatic nerve. Well, there's and it surely works. Becoming proactive by strengthening your heart muscles in addition to extending encourage muscle tissues, putting them into very good condition, helps encourage the majority of one's own weight and eliminates stress or injury related back pain.

Look, i am not talking about developing six-pack muscles . What i am speaking about is clearly basic conditioning; strengthening and conditioning the ab muscles, the obliques, hip adductors and abductors and hip flexors at the exact minimum combined side stretching hamstrings and in addition the muscles at the base is all that's required to reduce overtraining or, even if it occurs, to accelerate recovery at the fantastic bulk of cases. The purpose is it is the center which enables one to drift up on two-legs, to flex in addition to twist, so to sit readily, to lift to complete those activities which make you human. Caring for the critical muscle band has to be a top priority.

In case your goal would be to protect against the occurrence of menstruation afterward employed by 2-3 weeks using a fitness expert on developing a easy routine for your center is a fantastic idea. The workouts to the back and heart can be specific and also there are a great deal of muscles included. Attempting to generate a schedule by yourself can do more damage while in the future compared to just good. For certain, in the event that you presently have back pain then speak with your doctor and receive a referral to a physical therapist who will help you through the very ideal workout routine for relieving your discomfort. In a nutshell, do not make an effort to take care of your spine by yourself. Search expert guidance as it really is that essential.

No matter if you're performing exercises to state that the heart so as to relieve chronic back pain, then it's necessary to get them on the normal basis. If your objective is clearly pain relief, then you ought to achieve your exercises even in the event that you're damaging. Why is it conducive is your data that conditioning and strengthening the true core reduces your recovery period somewhat? The additional bonus of quitting a recurrence of this sciatica is really a long-term incentive based in the own effort.

When performing exercises for sciatica start off at a traditional manner. There's not any requirement to test to do everything simultaneously. Since your heart gets more sturdy add many walking, mowing the lawn, cardio and swimming in case you have a mind to achieve that. A powerful core supplies you with options which you cannot create whenever your heart has gone outside of illness.

All these days many caregivers recommend exercises for sciatica. Actually, the absolute best caregivers will supply you with a special, customized exercise program built round the root reason behind one's own sciatica. The goal of the exercise is twofold. Firstly, to relieve the instantaneous short term sciatic pain and second to construct your strength and state to protect against some future flare-ups of sciatica.

Even though most peoples first urge is to simply take with their own bed when struck sciatica, anything outside a few days mattress rest really does more damage than good. The shortage of movement is awful to the joints and the bones which donate to your own esophagus and will result in distress and lack of conditioning, and which subsequently may cause future traumas and much more annoyance.

When i said earlier in the day, ideally your work out regime will be tailored especially to your inherent problem that resulted in the sciatica. However, almost any app for prevention and relief of sciatica could incorporate these elements.

Stretches: stretching of these essential muscles within the field is very important; this can even boost the freedom of the joints and ligaments. You need to focus on this hamstring, the muscles behind your thighs, and also the piriformis muscle, which then runs throughout the buttocks. The stretches in many cases are removed from yoga and consuming full dismissed yoga is an advantage to all thoracic victims.

Core strengthening: the heart muscles of the spine and gut have to be strong as you possibly can in whoever has suffered any kind of spine problem. When there's a fault with the backbone, powerful heart muscles may help encourage that weakness. Once more yoga exercises are all good, but many physiotherapists urge pilates and also a lot of core-strengthening can be accomplished using a gym ball, fit ball or even swiss-ball. Which can be the exact same task, however, understood by an assortment of titles.

Aerobic exercise: this may aid with overall fitness, endurance and strength. However, you are going to wish to avert any superior impact exercise which can nourish the spine and cause you further problems. Swimming and walking would be ideal. The generally accepted target for walking will be usually to be in a position to reach 3 kilometers (5 kms) each day in a lively pace. But make sure you gradually develop for the when it's not used for you.

Form: " it nearly goes without saying, but you should be confident you are doing exactly the exercises properly, in proper shape. If you can cause further issues on the spine and sciatic nerve-wracking. If you've got somebody instruction you originally and viewing your own form. If that isn't possible, make certain that you follow some directions and diagrams into the correspondence.

Effective sciatica nerve treatment

I personally might love to supply you with the signs of sciatica. In this way you're going to have the ability to be aware of in case you've got it. Afterward, i will follow what the majority of individuals do to treatments. Finally, i will provide you an extra treatment others do - that's come to be the best and safe treatment for carry.

Sciatica occurs whenever there's aggravation to the thoracic nerve whenever there's degeneration of the low thoracic disks. When the disks are all worn, then the bone of the vertebra pinches the guts. Once the vertebrae is out of alignment that the manhood at which the guts is gets pinched.

From the gluteus maximus (buttocks) there's a muscle known as the piriformis. The thoracic should put under your muscle. But, there are instances when it really is finished the piriformis, also, on infrequent occasions, cut through the muscle.

Throughout improper diet that's mostly acidic rather than alkaline, there's a shortage of calcium at the disks. The disks also get there or stretchable might be described as a prolapsed disk.

In this degenerated say the border of these vertebrae just isn't eloquent and flat however, "teeth-like". Together with your spine out of alignment, there's a pull the piriformis. While this occurs, the piriformis muscle can pinch and then irritate nerve.

The pain could begin from the buttocks or it might stretch the leg down entirely into the heels. If you're experiencing this sort of pain, then you probably have time consuming.

A number of the feeling you might happen are: tingling, burning, tingling sensation at the leg and thigh. The condition can be so debilitating it gets it tough to walk

Most people picked a debilitating surgery in their own vertebrae but in accordance with dr. James Weinstein, a professor of orthopedic surgery in Dartmouth university, maintained a surgery isn't powerful. His analysis had been based on 2000 patients who'd ruptured disks and contrasted to people have been medicated nonsurgically.

Some people today assert that self-improvement works in families, it doesn't. Why is it seem that it works in families could be the exact identical way of life? When eating customs are identical, and that they truly are for huge numbers of men and women, it contributes to the "same cause and effect."

There are approximately 300,000 Americans who experience a surgery in their own vertebrae. Thus, in consequence, in line with dr. Weinstein, they're better than people that cope with sciatica in different ways.

Who will be most probably influenced?

People between the ages of 25-45 really have a issue using their vertebrae. Early correction of their vertebrae and appointment on life styles would be your better prevention for sciatica.

The sciatic nerve could be the largest from the body therefore that it mustn't looked within treatment. The aggravation is normally happened as a consequence of the misalignment of the vertebrae. Someone could get their bottoms out of alignment, not comprehend it suffer some pain - at early phases. For that reason, individuals have a tendency to dismiss a checkup.

A side from operation, a frequent kind of treatment is drugs, specifically, pain killers. Painkillers are awful on the kidneys and also, needless to say, it will not arrive at the explanation for the pain.

Some alternative treatments

To get better choices to this treatment of sciatic you can find lots of alternatives.

Eat a foods full of garlic, garlic, ginger and kelp. These herbs are referred to as anti-inflammatory.

Drink 68 glasses of plain water that's been filtered. This will avoid muscle cramps. You can't rely on coffee, tea and beverages as plain water whenever you're calculating your 6 8 drinks. This will look after the stiffness and stiffness related to sciatica.

Exercise is yet still another fantastic option. Specifically, a fitness in which you increase up your knees to your chest area. Good stretching of these thighs is effective, too.

Finally, lots of men and women that have sciatica will go to a professional of quantum-touch. Some physicians and osteopaths are currently incorporating this therapy inside their own practice. This treatment only entails a mild touch of their palms within the affected region and total treatment is preferred with most customers later one session.

Benefits of exercise for people with sciatica

Acute sciatic nerve pain may appear to be ineffective occasionally, therefore that I discovered ways to repair my sciatica. To get started using for a long time i would like to work with a heating system to use to relieve the pain however, once i removed heat the pain was there as awful or a few times worse. I then learned this, to repair my burnout, " i have to happen to be using icepacks for twenty five minutes every a couple of hours (this helped manner more compared to warmth) and followed with exercises intended to extend back and forth the pain which has been running down my thighs into the back, that really help hasten the healing procedure.

Should you be afflicted by acute back pain which runs down your buttocks, thighs and all of the way to your feet, then odds are that you suffer from sciatica. If you really don't understand what this really is, it's pain from the digestive tract being pinched damaged or using pressure placed onto it in many diverse sources.

Once i unearthed my spine pain was a result of a pinched sciatic nerve i began to search for means to repair my sciatica by understanding exactly what the guts was where it had been located within my physique. The sciatic nerve is upper nerve in our bodies, which begins from the spinal cord and also goes throughout the vertebrae and disks of the spinal cord down throughout the buttock down the thighs all of the way to your feet, why your feet sometimes tingle or feel helpless as well when undergo intense sciatica.

Now let us take a look at a few of things which cause sciatic nerve pain and damage:

- improper lifting of heavy items (here really is actually the top reason for this nerve damage)
- rust of the back because of aging
- pinching of the nerve because back injury such like, herniated or smashed disks
- degenerative disk disease
- pressure in the nerve from nerves swelling or swelling as a result of a busted piriformis muscle (this muscular is lean and attaches to the lower back runs down the buttocks and attaches into the thighbone, the sciatic nerve works beneath this muscle) this popularly called piriformis syndrome
- growing tumors in the backbone in the region of the nerve putting strain onto it
- a misaligned back

Knowing what exactly the guts is and where it's located caused it to be simpler for me personally to discover strategies to repair my sciatica, like i mentioned earlier in the day heat was the incorrect means to alleviate the pain, also perhaps not exercising which extended and concentrated the pain left the pain persist more. Once i began itself treatments that i came across within a e book referred to as "sciatica self-maintenance" i discovered that i relieve the pain faster and keep it from recurring in the foreseeable future. On certain occasions i discovered this to repair my toenails demanded a physician to re align the spine to relieve the strain on the guts afterward, with the correct exercises that i really could continue to keep the spine in alignment and block the sciatica from coming.

Yoga exercises

Who's wouldn't normally like to find yoga at no cost? Exactly like every one, you too could be enthusiastic about this way collection of free yoga exercises which are meant only for you! All these yoga practice will teach you on the best way best to exercise yoga; you simply must follow the directions carefully with full confidence.

Ashtanga yoga is really a string of unique kinds of exercises that ought to be practiced regularly to enhance somebody's health. Exercising raises the critical stream of energy and supplies a reassurance. The absolutely free exercises listed here are only different poses that will need to become practiced properly.

Yoga is additionally a method of alive. It features performing daily routine tasks at a normal period regular. Consider the habit of getting up in the daytime. In yoga, the everyday routine starts with the a predetermined procedure of exercise regular in three different points; original, japa significance knocking a few headline over and up to keep up exactly the exact comprehension; secondly, study by reading a few yoga programs; and next, meditation that ought to really be performed in a predetermined period in a predetermined place regular.

The initial present of these absolutely free yoga exercises needs to function as that the corpse pose, and also be replicated between other asana (yoga poses) so that as your last comfort. This present looks easy and it's really quite fine too. However, it ought to be useful for a lot more than just relaxing. You ought to utilize this particular pose for meditation when allowing the mind to obtain relax and strength.

Start those yoga exercises with a warmup exercises to relax and prepare your muscles to the upcoming exercises. After warm you up can carry out the shoulder lifts the natural after exercise and also a person's attention, and this can enhance your eyesight and protect against fatigue. For the upcoming exercises you may practice sun salutation that'll extend all of your body tissues, this to organize for the far harder exercises. Attempt also leg lift, that'll tone your leg muscles, so providing you with longer endurance and improved flexibility; mind rack posture is also decent for resting several of one's organs like heart.

As soon as you prepare your body and mind for longer challenging yoga practice, begin in the next manner.

Start with the bridge along with plough presents; this can improve your back's endurance. Initially, you might find it tough to reach the last position. However, with exercise you'll have the ability to accomplish this"asana". In the beginning you won't have the capacity to execute it but remember it is vital that you attempt and make it to the ideal location and train your own body to finally reach the absolutely balanced posture.

Later this pose, try out the forward bend present to excite the nervous system. Afterward it's possible to attempt the fish present, it strengthens the torso lungs and muscles.

Next pose is known as cobra pose. Women who have problems with degenerative issues might try out the cobra present, it arouses the pelvic and lower abdominal region, improving the flow and massaging the body organs.

Should you want to reinforce the back, then you definitely need to try out the locust pose. Locust pose is known to help prevent constipation.

The bow is just still another present to assist your spine area stay powerful and flexible at precisely the exact same period along with abdominal fat my additionally be reduced when the proper diet is put on. Furthering this yoga practice you are able to try out the half twist pose for the spines.

Breathing is an extremely essential aspect in practicing yoga. You're able to learn appropriate method of breathing and enhance it by practicing exactly the crow pose. With this particular present, you are able to better your arm and joints stamina too. Afterward it is possible to try out the hands to foot pose and also the triangle. This pose necessitates the strength and flexibility.

At the end of most of these yoga exercise exercises; be certain you do the corpse present to recover any energy that's been lost throughout these totally free yoga practice also to offer rest to the entire body.

You are able to decide to try these completely free yoga exercises by one and watch for yourself that one's work the right for you personally. Knowing the poses which benefit you, only ensure you usually do not over stretch yourself into doing those exercises also that you observe exactly the exact same pair of exercises regularly.

Should you are considering taking a sort of practice with the purpose of creating yourself feel and look far better that you have to give very serious thought to yoga.

Yoga works in your human body and mind and its results is understood in lots of diverse aspects - within our own bodies, their own health insurance and the way they look, and on our heads - how we view the planet.

Therefore just how do yoga exercises change from other kinds of exercise?

Yoga exercises, also called asanas or postures, are put on the full body of the body. Alternatively,

Lots of other workout regimes really are a sort of technology placed on the muscles of their human body. Which usually means that yoga exercises are more worried about more than simply the shallow growth of muscles. The bearings utilized in yoga exercises have a tendency to normalize the purposes of the full organism.

The advantage of yoga exercises is they could modulate the involuntary processes of respiration and help the flow and digestion, elimination and metabolism etc. The exercises also function to impact the working of the glands and glands, in addition to the nervous system and also your head. This outcome is reached by doing heavy breathing as your system is put into a variety of postures. Every one of those yoga exercises creates an alternative totality from the connection that is functional inside the organism.

Thus, yoga can influence person physically, emotionally, morally and emotionally. Yoga highlights the doctrine of exercise. Under its training experiences a feeling of awakening. Each one's abilities are more heightened, and yet one accomplishes equilibrium and endurance through these aerobic exercises, some of which are modeled following the movements of different

Creatures. In aerobic exercises, comfort is educated as a art, breathing for being a science, and emotional control of your human body for a way of harmonizing the body, mind, and soul.

The advanced stages of yoga require several years of special preparation-practices. Now's manner of living, its pace and environment, imply this is tricky to realize. But, practicing yoga, yoga and heavy breathing and relaxation methods, with some of the period dedicated to meditation and concentration is some thing

Everyone could reach.

Yoga exercises may have a beneficial impact on those that suffer from illness or disease. Whilst it isn't ready to cure those matters, practicing yoga may implies that obstacles and impurities have been removed to ensure nature may do its curative work.

Therefore, if you're searching for a sort of exercise is effective favorably on your system and mind, and also something which is relatively simple to squeeze in to a daily routine then not consume exercises. The expanding prevalence of yoga exercises ensures you will likely locate a yoga center or some gymnasium that provides local classes in your town. If, nevertheless, you don't need enough time for you to attend classes you'll find lots of novels and dvd's on aerobic exercises, which means that you may perform it in your home at some period if it's suitable for you personally.

Within just a day or two of performing yoga exercises it's likely to come to feel revitalized as well as more healthy. Continued training of yoga exercises may make us fitter and more joyful.

The ideal in indian conventional kind of exercising is meditation that can supply a helpful way by that to boost your brain and the soul within and adds essential strength to your individual's human body and it all needs to gain from yoga will be really to master about the appropriate bearings in addition to methods of breathing. Ostensibly, everyone may do yoga practice provided that they have a very yoga mat and also actually, should they ensure selecting the suitable yoga mat, then they also are able to enjoy greater and a lot more comfortable at the exact same time as relaxing cycling practice.

Earlier you choose a particular yoga practice mat tote it pays to you to have a look at the different available yoga exercises mats and also the truth is, choosing a eco-yoga physical exercise mat is likely to soon be wise since the one that's surely built from pvc will place your health in danger and so needs to be avoided because a wonderful bargain as you possibly can.

One in the accessories that are essential to save your mat is truly a yoga mat tote which also helps you take your yoga mat together with you where you move. In reality, the better yoga mats could be folded along with wrapped and those are able to be placed within a yoga mat tote and performed with you too as useful for keeping your yoga exercises mat whilst it isn't being used.

An excellent yoga mat tote should be capable of carrying out a significant yoga mat which can measure up to hundred inches and additionally the yoga mat tote is good fitted to carrying along on your own journeys plus in addition, it helps assure the mat remains comfy and is protected from the weather and naturally, out of dirt.

You are able to find quite a-few diverse styles from which to choose if it concerns a superb yoga mat tote and the one which you opt for will be dependent on the size at precisely the exact same period as fabric employed and depends upon its layouts and you'll discover also various models for you to elect choose pick from. The simple truth is that it's rather typical to run into that yoga practice mat totes are made from silk and sometimes cotton whereas people manufactured out of jute as well as oftentimes velvet may also be rather well-known.

You want to create sure the yoga exercises mat tote that you want on buying is lasting plus it needs to be hardy enough to resist normal damage and in addition, it might likewise encourage to have a very yoga mat tote that's watertight, also for everyone these features, a handbag made from cotton will probably soon be most suitable.

If it concerns a yoga mat handbag constructed from lace or silk, they'll generally have cotton liner (thick) which contributes to their durability too as durability and several have very interesting patterns and comprise vibrant colors too as possess brilliant textures and are appropriate to people that need something out in your standard.

Yoga exercises would be the perfect way to spare your mind also to focus heavily. As soon as you've seen a stressful situation, the thoughts, body and soul is worn outside and exhausted. The reason of them may possibly have been out of the interaction with different people or something which have resulted in a pity, anger, melancholy and disappointment in you personally. These feelings generated out of those circumstances needs to be published so you may live a more joyful life. 1 effective method and also way expressing your own outpoured feelings and feelings is by simply doing yoga exercises. Once you truly feel like crying aloud or breaking the tv, you're able to as an alternative release your anxiety through yoga exercises which can be effective and beneficial. Such a plan has functioned in lots of ways for diverse men and women. People of us who do not find sufficient time for themselves may perform yoga exercises as a way to relieve themselves. Sometimes, work has captured us up so closely we do not find time for you to curl up and state ourselves. Yoga exercises are among the better remedies for this issue. Yoga exercises might also be implemented and heard from school. There are a number of sessions offering yoga clinics. The exercises you'll see in school might be performed in your home. In reality, you are able to learn a few yoga exercises in home by yourself. You are only going to need to desire a tv and a videotape. The tape reveals the following steps and steps for each yoga practice. Throughout a weary and heavy daytime, you also may set just a small commitment and time in doing aerobic exercises. Also bear in mind that in doing yoga, then you will have to be persistent in practicing the exercises in order it will soon take effect and you'll find over time developments in your own entire body. After doing the yoga exercises, then you ought to curl up for the consequence of those positions occur place. This way, your system will collect the outcomes. Before doing the yoga exercises, then you ought to lay at a relaxed posture which means that you may focus well and never be diverted by outside forces. You won't feel discomfort or pain too. Yoga exercises may be done anytime of the time provided that you're free. Even though it selects virtually no moment, still, the very best time to clinic it really is each daytime. Before eating your breakfast, then your mind is dependent upon its condition of calmness and clear of distractions. This really may be the best time to accomplish exercises. Before doing the exercises, make certain the heart is ready. It ought not feel any self or pain. It's crucial to maintain a fantastic center which means your brain can get the job done well. The right spot to accomplish your yoga exercises would be a silent location. It ought to be well ventilated and free of most of disagreeable things as well as smell. You ought to be liberated of all probable distractions. Keeping a fantastic tummy can be crucial therefore you may feel well along with your gastrointestinal tract answers accurately. What you ought to do is to drain your intestines and clean your noses. You ought to stay fit and clean. Now you have obviously understood the critical reminders, then you can begin your yoga exercises and work out your way.

Yoga is among the exercises which have boundless health and fitness benefits; by the robust and elastic body, a calm mind, a luminous beautiful skin, fat reduction for healing. It gives immense benefits which not only joins your system, but additionally boosts your head in addition to the breathing strategy. It compels stability and leaves your life more serene, happier and fulfilling.

Routine yoga training will give you with all around fitness center. This suggests you won't you should be getting physically healthy; however, you'll also be receiving mentally and mentally fit throughout the exercises. That is authorized by different exercises such as positions, breathing methods and meditation which yoga comprises.

Now you can even shed weight with yoga in the event that you're too heavy or in the event that you only need to drop some weight to better the physique. Once you take out yoga clinics, you'll begin becoming sensitive regarding the foods which you will likely be giving your entire body and the perfect time you'll be carrying foods. While doing so, you'll be keeping tabs on your own weight reduction.

Yoga methods can allow you to relieve stress that collects daily. With only a couple of minutes of yoga, then you will really feel liberated on the own body in addition to mind from some other stress which you may be going right through. The yoga poses, meditation and also the breathing processes can assist you to overcome tension and melancholy. In an advanced level yoga grade, it is possible to even utilize yoga exercises to detoxing your system and de-stressing mind.

Still another health advantage you can receive from yoga exercises will be inner peace. When a few folks desire inner serenity, they see quite places rich in natural magnificence.

Nonetheless, it's also great to be aware you could experience inner peace anywhere you might be and in any given moment. As an example, doing yoga exercises on your house will be able to assist you to get the inner peace that's available right in it. You do not necessarily need to attend a particular spot to have it. Inner-peace is quite essential in calming a troubled mind.

Now you may also gain from improved resistance if you execute routine exercises. For the body to get the job done well, your body mind and soul require to blend together. When there was an irregularity within your system, your head is going to be influenced inducing to experience guilt or unpleasantness. The yoga poses can also enable you to strengthen your muscles and also massage your own muscles. Besides relieving you in stress, breathing and meditation techniques may even enhance your own immunity.

Routine Pilates exercises can make the own body to own better posture and flexibility. Should you really miss a human body that's strong, flexible and supple, the trick is to add yoga in your ordinary routine. The own body tissues will be elongated and tone plus they'll become stronger. The own body posture once you stand, sit, sleep or walk will probably be made better. In the event that you will often possess human body aches because of incorrect position, yoga methods may assist you to overcome them.

Now you may likewise feel pumped up with energy in the event you maintain routine exercises. Should you feel tired out by the ending of your afternoon, or you also detect taking out multiple activities to become quite tiring, a couple minutes of exercising every day will make you feeling lively and fresh daily. Throughout your afternoon, you'll likely be refreshed and prepared to execute those activities of daily.

When you execute yoga exercises frequently, and you will

establish greater intuition. Meditation can enhance your instinctive capability and permit one to comprehend cheaply what ought to be achieved, how it has to be achieved and exactly what period it has to be carried out. This can allow you to yield very good outcomes or boost your performance in your everyday pursuits.

In early India, yoga has been a method of living that comprised moral, moral, religious, and physiological components. Postures (asana) were also an essential, but tiny sector of the early clinic. Today, a lot of men and women make use of the word "yoga" to mean a certain sort of physical exercise, even while being totally oblivious of its own spiritual part, making the present-day model of meditation a shadow of its former self. Some classes wind without a time spent from the worthiness of pranayama, relaxation, or meditation.

To put it yet another way, the vital yoga mat, utilized in today's exercise variant, could just be needed to get a modest part of a genuine yoga clinic. As stated by maharishi Patanjali's writings, at the yoga sutras, asana is simply among eight limbs over yogic philosophy - most which can be utilized to organize for the greatest marriage of someone's inner intellect together with worldwide comprehension. As stated by proponents of conventional yoga, it's not possible to accomplish enlightenment simply by doing a bodily practice, even when a person practices the very complex postures.

In addition to providing a twisted view of this original clinic, contemporary yoga was sidetracked and used as a procedure to market popularity and sell pictures to people. This consists of personal stardom, and any such thing from correct organic mats, for high priced high style accessories and clothing. While this isn't inherently bad whatsoever, it scarcely looks like the humble way of life, and unwavering dedication, of those numerous sages, who retained yoga living for generations throughout Sanskrit texts and oral teachings. When yogic teachings gained worldwide awareness, it was just natural to modern yoga to simply take its own individuality.

This doesn't follow that the bodily exercises at modern meditation are poor or some less efficient compared to people at different tasks. In reality, asanas and leaks maybe more powerful than a number of different sorts of exercise. Studies have revealed that yoga movement improves physical health and fitness, help prevent illness, reduce depression and stress, reduce anxiety, promote comfort, and an overall awareness of wellbeing. Purists, however, could wonder if these fitness-based styles ought to really be called yoga.

The fact remains that few folks in the 21stcentury, are most likely to devote long intervals at ashrams because apprentices, meditating, and living the life span of some conventional yogi. In reality, a little bit of yoga is definitely greater than no yoga in any way. If modern yoga exercises is really helping create a more healthy and more peaceful society, also reducing the amazing price of health care bills, it's magic in itself.

Still another issue with modern yoga is that the significantly confusing actuality that a few folks think it to be counterproductive with their own religious beliefs or opinion systems. Meditation is a life style, not just a religion. Yoga doesn't discriminate. It will not look to hinder human beliefs or rationale, and anybody is welcome to appreciate its benefits. Afterall, who can assert with a fitter, happier, more peaceful planet?

The exercise is imagined to loosen the central nervous system and also stabilize the whole human body, mind, and soul. It's thought with its own enthusiasts to steer clear of certain ailments.

Doing this type of exercise usually help make the human body's immune mechanisms strong assisting your own body to be in a position to manage lots of disorders like annoyance, fatigue and so forth. The curative rate of a personal accident or only a wound can be additionally enhanced. In addition, yoga practice was employed to lessen hyper tension degrees, reduce stress, and boost coordination, endurance, attention, sleeping, and food digestion. Medical professionals along with scientists have been researching latest the huge benefits of exercising regularly. Studies demonstrate that it might potentially decrease the signs of many popular and sometimes life-threatening disorders including arthritis, arteriosclerosis, acute fatigue, diabetes, obesity, aids, asthma attack along with weight loss issues.

Together with treating disorders, yoga practice is presently one among the choices for drugs. Together with yoga exercises like a combination of physical exercises, breathing exercises, and meditation, it turns to a specially effective type of physical activity for people that have certain medical difficulties. For anyone who have cardiovascular disease, various studies have proven yoga practice to aid people young and old. In particular, the exercise appears to enhance cardiovascular disease in lots of ways, including controlling elevated blood pressure rates and increasing immunity to emotional stress. Scientific tests made at yoga establishments in india have recorded impressive success in relieving asthma. Additionally, it has been proven that asthma conditions can normally be prevented by way of yoga courses without turning into medicinal drugs. Yoga can be thought to decrease pain by helping the brain's pain center regulates the gate-controlling system found in the back and also the release of natural pain killers in the physique. Cardiovascular exercises utilized in yoga additionally can reduce strain. Considering the fact that muscles have a tendency to curl up once you breathe, widening time of exhalation can help provide comfort decreasing strain. Recognizing breathing helps to acquire calmer, less fast respiration and help with comfort and pain control. Yoga has got the chance to buffer against the damaging impact of physiological self-objectification also to build up embodiment and wellbeing.

Moreover, the practice was broadly studied as a way in lowering (and occasionally remove) many cardiovascular risks. A number of these unwanted side effects include lower the circulation of blood, renal system failure, menopausal failure, as well as blindness. Many researchers believe practicing yoga and with daily aid services and products on a frequent basis might help stimulate blood circulation and massage tissues, which regularly can offer long-term bodily advantages to people fighting diabetes. In addition, the practice of yoga may provide long-term benefits for those who have diabetes because this was ascertained to decrease sugar levels, obtaining a fantastic result on every kind of diabetes, including type 1 and type 2 diabetes.

Yoga exercise is actually the very best medicine for several sort of health issues and also a very excellent refresher of individual brain, body and soul. It helps to get a person emotionally and emotionally productive. Consequently, everyone should start performing yoga exercise often to remain healthy and fit to very existence.

Acute sciatic nerve pain may appear to be ineffective occasionally, therefore that i discovered ways to repair my sciatica. To get started using for a long time i would like to work with a heating system to use to relieve the pain however, once i removed heat the pain was there as awful or a few times worse. I then learned this, to repair my burnout, " i have to happen to be using icepacks for twenty five minutes every a couple of hours (this helped manner more compared to warmth) and followed with exercises intended to extend back and forth the pain which has been running down my thighs into the back, that really help hasten the healing procedure.

Should you be afflicted by acute back pain which runs down your buttocks, thighs and all of the way to your feet, then odds are that you suffer from sciatica. If you really don't understand what this really is, it's pain from the digestive tract being pinched damaged or using pressure placed onto it in many diverse sources.

Once i unearthed my spine pain was a result of a pinched sciatic nerve i began to search for means to repair my sciatica by understanding exactly what the guts was where it had been located within my physique. The sciatic nerve is upper nerve in our bodies, which begins from the spinal cord and also goes throughout the vertebrae and disks of the spinal cord down throughout the buttock down the thighs all of the way to your feet, why your feet sometimes tingle or feel helpless as well when undergo intense sciatica.

Now let us take a look at a few of things which cause sciatic nerve pain and damage:

- improper lifting of heavy items (here really is actually the top reason for this nerve damage)
- rust of the back because of aging
- pinching of the nerve because back injury such like, herniated or smashed disks
- degenerative disk disease
- pressure in the nerve from nerves swelling or swelling as a result of a busted piriformis muscle (this muscular is lean and attaches to the lower back runs down the buttocks and attaches into the thighbone, the sciatic nerve works beneath this muscle) this popularly called piriformis syndrome

- growing tumors in the backbone in the region of the nerve putting strain onto it
- a misaligned back

Knowing what exactly the guts is and where it's located caused it to be simpler for me personally to discover strategies to repair my sciatica, like i mentioned earlier in the day heat was the incorrect means to alleviate the pain, also perhaps not exercising which extended and concentrated the pain left the pain persist more. Once I began itself treatments that i came across within a e book referred to as "sciatica self-maintenance" I discovered that i relieve the pain faster and keep it from recurring in the foreseeable future. On certain occasions I discovered this to repair my toenails demanded a physician to re align the spine to relieve the strain on the guts afterward, with the correct exercises that i really could continue to keep the spine in alignment and block the sciatica from coming.

Yoga exercises

Who's wouldn't normally like to find yoga at no cost? Exactly like every one, you too could be enthusiastic about this way collection of free yoga exercises which are meant only for you! All these yoga practice will teach you on the best way best to exercise yoga; you simply must follow the directions carefully with full confidence.

Ashtanga yoga is really a string of unique kinds of exercises that ought to be practiced regularly to enhance somebody's health. Exercising raises the critical stream of energy and supplies a reassurance. The absolutely free exercises listed here are only different poses that will need to become practiced properly.

Yoga is additionally a method of alive. It features performing daily routine tasks at a normal period regular. Consider the habit of getting up in the daytime. In yoga, the everyday routine starts with the a predetermined procedure of exercise regular in three different points; original, japa significance knocking a few headline over and up to keep up exactly the exact comprehension; secondly, study by reading a few yoga programs; and next, meditation that ought to really be performed in a predetermined period in a predetermined place regular.

The initial present of these absolutely free yoga exercises needs to function as that the corpse pose, and also be replicated between other asana (yoga poses) so that as your last comfort. This present looks easy and it's really quite fine too. However, it ought to be useful for a lot more than just relaxing. You ought to utilize this particular pose for meditation when allowing the mind to obtain relax and strength.

Start those yoga exercises with an warmup exercises to relax and prepare your muscles to the upcoming exercises. After warm you up can carry out the shoulder lifts the natural after exercise and also a person's attention, and this can enhance your eyesight and protect against fatigue. For the upcoming exercises you may practice sun salutation that'll extend all of your body tissues, this to organize for the far harder exercises. Attempt also leg lift, that'll tone your leg muscles, so providing you with longer endurance and improved flexibility; mind rack posture is also decent for resting several of one's organs like heart.

As soon as you prepare your body and mind for longer challenging yoga practice, begin in the next manner.

Start with the bridge along with plough presents; this can improve your back's endurance. Initially, you might find it tough to reach the last position. However, with exercise you'll have the ability to accomplish this "asana". In the beginning you won't have the capacity to execute it but remember it is vital that you attempt and make it to the ideal location and train your own body to finally reach the absolutely balanced posture.

Later this pose, try out the forward bend present to excite the nervous system. Afterward it's possible to attempt the fish present, it strengthens the torso lungs and muscles.

Next pose is known as cobra pose. Women who have problems with degenerative issues might try out the cobra present, it arouses the pelvic and lower abdominal region, improving the flow and massaging the body organs.

Should you want to reinforce the back, then you definitely need to try out the locust pose. Locust pose is known to help prevent constipation.

The bow is just still another present to assist your spine area stay powerful and flexible at precisely the exact same period along with abdominal fat my additionally be reduced when the proper diet is put on. Furthering this yoga practice you are able to try out the half twist pose for the spines.

Breathing is an extremely essential aspect in practicing yoga. You're able to learn appropriate method of breathing and enhance it by practicing exactly the crow pose. With this particular present, you are able to better your arm and joints stamina too. Afterward it is possible to try out the hands to foot pose and also the triangle. This pose necessitates the strength and flexibility.

At the end of most of these yoga exercise exercises; be certain you do the corpse present to recover any energy that's been lost throughout these totally free yoga practice also to offer rest to the entire body.

You are able to decide to try these completely free yoga exercises by one and watch for yourself that one's work the right for you personally. Knowing the poses which benefit you, only ensure you usually do not over stretch yourself into doing those exercises also that you observe exactly the exact same pair of exercises regularly.

Should you are considering taking a sort of practice with the purpose of creating yourself feel and look far better that you have to give very serious thought to yoga .

Yoga works in your human body and mind and its results is understood in lots of diverse aspects - within our own bodies, their own health insurance and the way they look, and on our heads - how we view the planet.

Therefore, just how do yoga exercises change from other kinds of exercise?

Yoga exercises, also called asanas or postures, are put on the full body of the body. Alternatively,

Lots of other workout regimes really are a sort of technology placed on the muscles of their human body. Which usually means that yoga exercises are more worried about more than simply the shallow growth of muscles. The bearings utilized in yoga exercises have a tendency to normalize the purposes of the full organism.

The advantage of yoga exercises is they could modulate the involuntary processes of respiration and help the flow and digestion, elimination and metabolism etc. The exercises also function to impact the working of the glands and glands, in addition to the nervous system and also your head. This outcome is reached by doing heavy breathing as your system is put into a variety of postures. Every one of those yoga exercises creates an alternative totality from the connection that is functional inside the organism.

Thus, yoga can influence person physically, emotionally, morally and emotionally. Yoga highlights the doctrine of exercise. Under its training experiences a feeling of awakening. Each one's abilities are more heightened, and yet one accomplishes equilibrium and endurance through these aerobic exercises, some of which are modeled following the movements of different

Creatures. In aerobic exercises, comfort is educated as a art, breathing for being a science, and emotional control of your human body for a way of harmonizing the body, mind, and soul.

The advanced stages of yoga require several years of special preparation-practices. Now's manner of living, its pace and environment, imply this is tricky to realize. But, practicing yoga, yoga and heavy breathing and relaxation methods, with some of the period dedicated to meditation and concentration is some thing

Everyone could reach.

Yoga exercises may have a beneficial impact on those that suffer from illness or disease. Whilst it isn't ready to cure those matters, practicing yoga may implies that obstacles and impurities have been removed to ensure nature may do its curative work.

Therefore, if you're searching for a sort of exercise is effective favorably on your system and mind, and also something which is relatively simple to squeeze in to a daily routine then not consume exercises. The expanding prevalence of yoga exercises ensures you will likely locate a yoga center or some gymnasium that provides local classes in your town. If, nevertheless, you don't need enough time for you to attend classes you'll find lots of novels and dvd's on aerobic exercises, which means that you may perform it in your home at some period if it's suitable for you personally.

Within just a day or two of performing yoga exercises it's likely to come to feel revitalized as well as healthier. Continued training of yoga exercises may make us fitter and more joyful.

The ideal in Indian conventional kind of exercising is meditation that can supply a helpful way by that to boost your brain and the soul within and adds essential strength to your individual's human body and it all needs to gain from yoga will be really to master about the appropriate bearings in addition to methods of breathing. Ostensibly, everyone may do yoga practice provided that they have a very yoga mat and also actually, should they ensure selecting the suitable yoga mat, then they also are able to enjoy greater and a lot more comfortable at the exact same time as relaxing cycling practice.

Earlier you choose a particular yoga practice mat tote it pays to you to have a look at the different available yoga exercises mats and also the truth is, choosing a eco-yoga physical exercise mat is likely to soon be wise since the one that's surely built from pvc will place your health in danger and so needs to be avoided because a wonderful bargain as you possibly can.

One in the accessories that are essential to save your mat is truly a yoga mat tote which also helps you take your yoga mat together with you where you move. In reality, the better yoga mats could be folded along with wrapped and those are able to be placed within a yoga mat tote and performed with you too as useful for keeping your yoga exercises mat whilst it isn't being used.

An excellent yoga mat tote should be capable of carrying out a significant yoga mat which can measure up to hundred inches and additionally the yoga mat tote is good fitted to carrying along on your own journeys plus in addition, it helps assure the mat remains comfy and is protected from the weather and naturally, out of dirt.

You are able to find quite a-few diverse styles from which to choose if it concerns a superb yoga mat tote and the one which you opt for will be dependent on the size at precisely the exact same period as fabric employed and depends upon its layouts and you'll discover also various models for you to elect choose pick from. The simple truth isthat it's rather typical to run into that yoga practice mat totes are made from silk and sometimes cotton whereas people manufactured out of jute as well as oftentimes velvet may also be rather well-known.

You want to create sure the yoga exercises mat tote that you want on buying is lasting plus it needs to be hardy enough to resist normal damage and in addition, it might likewise encourage to have a very yoga mat tote that's watertight, also for everyone these features, a handbag made from cotton will probably soon be most suitable.

If it concerns a yoga mat handbag constructed from lace or silk, they'll generally have cotton liner (thick) which contributes to their durability too as durability and several have very interesting patterns and comprise vibrant colors too as possess brilliant textures and are appropriate to people that need something out in your standard.

Yoga exercises would be the perfect way to spare your mind also to focus heavily. As soon as you've seen a stressful situation, the thoughts, body and soul is worn outside and exhausted. The reason of them may possibly have been out of the interaction with different people or something which have resulted in a pity, anger, melancholy and disappointment in you personally. These feelings generated out of those circumstances needs to be published so you may live a more joyful life. 1 effective method and also way expressing your own outpoured feelings and feelings is by simply doing yoga exercises. Once you truly feel like crying aloud or breaking the tv, you're able to as an alternative release your anxiety through yoga exercises which can be effective and beneficial. Such a plan has functioned in lots of ways for diverse men and women. People of us who do not find sufficient time for themselves may perform yoga exercises as a way to relieve themselves. Sometimes, work has captured us up so closely we do not find time for you to curl up and state ourselves. Yoga exercises are among the better remedies for this issue. Yoga exercises might also be implemented and heard from school. There are a number of sessions offering yoga clinics. The exercises you'll see in school might be performed in your home. In reality, you are able to learn a few yoga exercises in home by yourself. You are only going to need to desire a tv and a videotape. The tape reveals the following steps and steps for each yoga practice. Throughout a weary and heavy daytime, you also may set just a small commitment and time in doing aerobic exercises. Also bear in mind that in doing yoga, then you will have to be persistent in practicing the exercises in order it will soon take effect and you'll find over time developments in your own entire body. After doing the yoga exercises, then you ought to curl up for the consequence of those positions occur place. This way, your system will collect the outcomes. Before doing the yoga exercises, then you ought to lay at a relaxed posture which means that you may focus well and never be diverted by outside forces. You won't feel discomfort or pain too. Yoga exercises may be done anytime of the time provided that you're free. Even though it selects virtually no moment, still, the very best time to clinic it really is each daytime. Before eating your breakfast, then your mind is dependent upon its condition of calmness and clear of distractions. This really may be the best time to accomplish exercises. Before doing the exercises, make certain the heart is ready. It ought not feel any self or pain. It's crucial to maintain a fantastic center which means your brain can get the job done well. The right spot to accomplish your yoga exercises would be a silent location. It ought to be well ventilated and free of most of disagreeable things as well as smell. You ought to be liberated of all probable distractions. Keeping a fantastic tummy can be crucial therefore you may feel well along with your gastrointestinal tract answers accurately. What you ought to do is to drain your intestines and clean your noses. You ought to stay fit and clean. Now you have obviously understood the critical reminders, then you can begin your yoga exercises and work out your way.

Yoga is among the exercises which have boundless health and fitness benefits; by the robust and elastic body, a calm mind, a luminous beautiful skin, fat reduction for healing. It gives immense benefits which not only joins your system, but additionally boosts your head in addition to the breathing strategy. It compels stability and leaves your life more serene, happier and fulfilling.

Routine yoga training will give you with all around fitness center. This suggests you won't you should be getting physically healthy; however you'll also be receiving mentally and mentally fit throughout the exercises. That is authorized by different exercises such as positions, breathing methods and meditation which yoga comprises.

Now you can even shed weight with yoga in the event that you're too heavy or in the event that you only need to drop some weight to better the physique. Once you take out yoga clinics, you'll begin becoming sensitive regarding the foods which you will likely be giving your entire body and the perfect time you'll be carrying foods. While doing so, you'll be keeping tabs on your own weight reduction.

Yoga methods can allow you to relieve stress that collects daily. With only a couple of minutes of yoga, then you will really feel liberated on the own body in addition to mind from some other stress which you may be going right through. The yoga poses, meditation and also the breathing processes can assist you to overcome tension and melancholy. In an advanced level yoga grade, it is possible to even utilize yoga exercises to detoxing your system and de-stressing mind.

Still another health advantage you can receive from yoga exercises will be inner peace. When a few folks desire inner serenity, they see quite places rich in natural magnificence. Nonetheless, it's also great to be aware you could experience inner peace anywhere you might be and in any given moment. As an example, doing yoga exercises on your house will be able to assist you to get the inner peace that's available right in it. You do not necessarily need to attend a particular spot to have it. Inner-peace is quite essential in calming a troubled mind.

Now you may also gain from improved resistance if you execute routine exercises. For the body to get the job done well, your bodymind and soul require to blend together. When there was an irregularity within your system, your head is going to be influenced inducing to experience guilt or unpleasantness. The yoga poses can also enable you to strengthen your muscles and also massage your own muscles. Besides relieving you in stress, breathing and meditation techniques may even enhance your own immunity.

Routine Pilates exercises can make the own body to own better posture and flexibility. Should you really miss a human body that's strong, flexible and supple, the trick is to add yoga in your ordinary routine. The own body tissues will be elongated and tone plus they'll become stronger. The own body posture once you stand, sit, sleep or walk will probably be made better. In the event that you will often possess human body aches because of incorrect position, yoga methods may assist you to overcome them.

Now you may likewise feel pumped up with energy in the event you maintain routine exercises. Should you feel tired out by the ending of your afternoon, or you also detect taking out multiple activities to become quite tiring, a couple minutes of exercising every day will make you feeling lively and fresh daily. Throughout your afternoon, you'll likely be refreshed and prepared to execute those activities of daily.

When you execute yoga exercises frequently, and you will establish greater intuition. Meditation can enhance your instinctive capability and permit one to comprehend cheaply what ought to be achieved, how it has to be achieved and exactly what period it has to be carried out. This can allow you to yield very good outcomes or boost your performance in your everyday pursuits.

In early India, yoga has been a method of living that comprised moral, moral, religious, and physiological components. Postures (asana) were also an essential, but tiny sector of the early clinic. Today, a lot of men and women make use of the word "yoga" to mean a certain sort of physical exercise, even while being totally oblivious of its own spiritual part, making the present-day model of meditation a shadow of its former self. Some classes wind without a time spent from the worthiness of pranayama, relaxation, or meditation.

To put it yet another way, the vital yoga mat, utilized in today's exercise variant, could just be needed to get a modest part of a genuine yoga clinic. As stated by maharishi Patanjali's writings, at the yoga sutras, asana is simply among eight limbs over yogic philosophy - most which can be utilized to organize for the greatest marriage of someone's inner intellect together with worldwide comprehension. As stated by proponents of conventional yoga, it's not possible to accomplish enlightenment simply by doing a bodily practice, even when a person practices the very complex postures.

In addition to providing a twisted view of this original clinic, contemporary yoga was sidetracked and used as a procedure to market popularity and sell pictures to people. This consists of personal stardom, and any such thing from correct organic mats, for high priced high style accessories and clothing. While this isn't inherently bad whatsoever, it scarcely looks like the humble way of life, and unwavering dedication, of those numerous sages, who retained yoga living for generations throughout Sanskrit texts and oral teachings. When yogic teachings gained worldwide awareness, it was just natural to modern yoga to simply take its own individuality.

This doesn't follow that the bodily exercises at modern meditation are poor or some less efficient compared to people at different tasks. In reality, asanas and leaks maybe more powerful than a number of different sorts of exercise. Studies have revealed that yoga movement improves physical health and fitness, help prevent illness, reduce depression and stress, reduce anxiety, promote comfort, and an overall awareness of wellbeing. Purists, however, could wonder if these fitness-based styles ought to really be called yoga.

The fact remains that few folks in the 21stcentury, are most likely to devote long intervals at ashrams because apprentices, meditating, and living the life span of some conventional yogi. In reality, a little bit of yoga is definitely greater than no yoga in any way. If modern yoga exercises is really helping create a more healthy and more peaceful society, also reducing the amazing price of health care bills, it's magic in itself.

Still another issue with modern yoga is that the significantly confusing actuality that a few folks think it to be counterproductive with their own religious beliefs or opinion systems. Meditation is a life style, not just a religion. Yoga doesn't discriminate. It will not look to hinder human beliefs or rationale, and anybody is welcome to appreciate its benefits. Afterall, who can assert with a fitter, happier, more peaceful planet?

The exercise is imagined to loosen the central nervous system and also stabilize the whole human body, mind, and soul. It's thought with its own enthusiasts to steer clear of certain ailments. Doing this type of exercise usually help make the human body's immune mechanisms strong assisting your own body to be in a position to manage lots of disorders like annoyance, fatigue and so forth. The curative rate of a personal accident or only a wound can be additionally enhanced. In addition, yoga practice was employed to lessen hyper tension degrees, reduce stress, and boost coordination, endurance, attention, sleeping, and food digestion. Medical professionals along with scientists have been researching latest the huge benefits of exercising regularly. Studies demonstrate that it might potentially decrease the signs of many popular and sometimes life-threatening disorders including arthritis, arteriosclerosis, acute fatigue, diabetes, obesity, aids, asthma attack along with weight loss issues.

Together with treating disorders, yoga practice is presently one among the choices for drugs. Together with yoga exercises like a combination of physical exercises, breathing exercises, and meditation, it turns to a especially effective type of physical activity for people that have certain medical difficulties. For anyone who have cardiovascular disease, various studies have proven yoga practice to aid people young and old. In particular, the exercise appears to enhance cardiovascular disease in lots of ways, including controlling elevated blood pressure rates and increasing immunity to emotional stress. Scientific tests made at yoga establishments in India have recorded impressive success in relieving asthma. Additionally, it has been proven that asthma conditions can normally be prevented by way of yoga courses without turning into medicinal drugs. Yoga can be thought to decrease pain by helping the brain's pain center regulates the gate-controlling system found in the back and also the release of natural pain killers in the physique. Cardiovascular exercises utilized in yoga additionally can reduce strain. Considering the fact that muscles have a tendency to curl up once you breathe, widening time of exhalation can help provide comfort decreasing strain. Recognizing breathing helps to acquire calmer, less fast respiration and help with comfort and pain control. Yoga has got the chance to buffer against the damaging impact of physiological self-objectification also to build up embodiment and wellbeing.

Moreover, the practice was broadly studied as a way in lowering (and occasionally remove) many cardiovascular risks. A number of these unwanted side effects include lower the circulation of blood, renal system failure, menopausal failure, as well as blindness. Many researchers believe practicing yoga and with daily aid services and products on a frequent basis might help stimulate blood circulation and massage tissues, which regularly can offer long-term bodily advantages to people fighting diabetes. In addition, the practice of yoga may provide long-term benefits for those who have diabetes because this was ascertained to decrease sugar levels, obtaining a fantastic result on every kind of diabetes, including type 1 and type 2 diabetes.

Yoga exercise is actually the very best medicine for several sort of health issues and also a very excellent refresher of individual brain, body and soul. It helps to get a person emotionally and emotionally productive. Consequently, everyone should start performing yoga exercise often to remain healthy and fit to very existence.

CHAPTER SIX

༭

Sciatica exercises for pain management

S ciatica anxiety can be tricky to live with, impacting every part of a sufferer's daily life. There are lots of alternatives for sciatica pain alleviation; it could be handled by inpatient home remedies, such as cold and hot therapy and physical exercise. Sciatica pain may be handled using drugs. In acute circumstances, pain may be relieved or handled using operation.

In the last, bed remainder was frequently suggested for patients suffering from pain. Nowadays, however, doctors and physical therapists equally are counseling against this clinic. As an alternative, a normal gentle exercise regime is advised. Targeted stretches, such as yoga methods, are also utilized to alleviate pain. Sciatica treatment may be gotten with cold and hot therapy in your home. Applying ice packs to the affected area offers treatment. Filled with warmth provides the muscles that are affected an opportunity to relaxand relieving strain over the compressed nerve and also relieving the pain that the victim feels.

Drug can be also a choice for sciatica pain alleviation. Sciatica pain is treated using a anti inflammatory medication like ibuprofen or codeine. In acute instances, cortisone shots might also be managed for temporary treatment. Sufferers must remember, nevertheless, why these drugs simply alleviate the annoyance. They usually do not heal the underlying problem.

In acute instances, sciatica sufferers may buy respite from

operation. If puberty is being brought on by a spinal trauma, like a slipped or herniated disc, surgery may alleviate the rear harm, and so the stress on the sciatic nerve. If you're having chronic gastrointestinal pain, then speak with your physician about what options may be ideal for you personally.

The best way can lyrica and sciatica link solely to another? Anxiety with sciatica can impair the usual lifetime and cause agonizing pain. It could and can restrict your ability to walk and the skill to proceed. Usually the pain is principally using a single side of their human anatomy. It's going to begin at the back and then proceed its way down the cool and all of the way to the feet.

Additionally, it is frequently abbreviated because of disorder in reality, lyrica and endometriosis really are a combination which helps relieve the chronic pain which could be a consequence of the compressed or pinched nerve or a irritation to the nerves. The therapy needed would all depend on what's causing the pinched nerve.

Lyrica and sciatica pain control is an extremely significant part the nerve procedure process. Any movement will probably lead to pain, and also the patient chooses to confine their movement due to the pain entailed. If they simply sit that is a lot easier than most of the annoyance. However, this may be dangerous and will lead to stiffness in the joints and muscles. And also this can lead to more pain and problems.

The secret to handling so, the trick to all other remedies for sciatica would be really exercise. Pain management is essential, but even thus the affected individual is preferred to sustain an inpatient workout regime.

Sciatica pain control is just one of the main facts to take into consideration when treating your own pain. People all over the globe suffer with plantar pain and also a few understand just how to manage it. Below are a number of ways which you may safely and effortlessly maintain your sciatica symptoms off.

One method to deal with your sciatica is through exercises and stretches. Even though these are extremely effective, few folks would follow on an everyday basis. It's imperative that you stay together with stretching which will work and throw off the ones which aren't. Attempt to accomplish your exercises and stretches regular, even when it's only for five full minutes. After a month or two or weeks, then you will realize a dramatic decline in pain. But do not end there. Regular you ought to be continuously exercising or extending, even when pain has escalated. This will reduce the possibility of one's pain coming back and with you reside with sedation again.

Still another method to deal with your sciatic pain is via therapy. Seeing a physical therapist in an everyday basis can reduce your symptoms, sometimes the initial moment. Even though this is often frustrating, it's extremely powerful. Going to the community physician and advocating seeing a physical therapist can be the starting place. As soon as you've discovered the one that's ideal for you, stay to this app. Establish certain goals for yourself and stay motivated. The further you're inclined to triumph, the faster that your result will likely be.

As you're able to easily see, there really are an assortment of means to aid in managing your own sciatica. Make sure you sick with whichever application that you proceed through and stay motivated. The trick is copying, the longer you elongate or view a therapist, the greater your odds will be for a fast and effortless recovery.

In case you're feeling pain in your own lower back when you bend or stretch also it melts to your thighs, you then could be undergoing sciatica. However, what exactly is sciatica? It's a pain symptom that caused the aggravation of the sciatic nerve. The pain usually begins at the low back and could stretch to the foot and calf based upon the affected nerve origin. Sciatica isn't just a disease alone but a symptom caused the other health illness. Individuals who're often afflicted with sciatica are afflicted by the herniated disk. One other element which directly impacts aggravation and swelling in the sciatic nerve produces the signs of sciatica.

The sciatic nerve is the largest nerve in your system. Its neural roots run in the thoracic back located at the low back stretching throughout the buttocks, shoulders and lower limb. If this nerve becomes irritated or inflamed it produces pain which looks such as a leg . It generates sitting nor standing difficult on account of the high level of pain it soothes. An average of the pain is aggravated after sitting, coughing or sneezing. Illness in severe puberty usually lasts for four to eight weeks plus reduces on a unique based upon the causative agent.

Sciatica is frequently brought on by the slipping of disks. It's normal in people between the ages of 30-50 partially as a result of aging. The overall damage of the encompassing muscular of the spine can readily be afflicted with any abrupt pressure on the discs. The discs function as a pillow of this bone at the low spine of course, whether or not it deteriorates can lead into the manifestation of puberty; the high degree of pain caused by sciatica fluctuates.

The compression of the thoracic nerve contributes to sciatica. After the disk slips or lumps, pain in the back is the initial symptom which is being shown. Its symptoms can include tingling sensation, numbness and tingling sense.

Diagnosis of sciatica normally comprises a comprehensive clinical assessment. In general, the physician explains the way a pain started and its own symptoms. Appropriate knowledge and comprehension are crucial to your affected individual to clearly comprehend what's sciatica and just how can this affect them. Your health care provider could also need to examine its symptoms and signs through a concrete examination. Physical exam can also help determine its origin to be in a position to offer a definite outlook. The evaluation can be also utilized to pin point the most nerves that are affected. Other evaluations like Xray and mri could be recommended for additional evaluation.

Ostensibly the most important objective of treatment for sciatica would be always to diminish pain, stiffness and increase freedom. The cure for sedation would ordinarily involve rehab, medical and surgery direction. If puberty happens untreated it may possibly result in a chronic illness and further complications. Intense sciatica illness usually goes off with good time and rest, with no necessity for surgery or some other medical direction. There are means to help stop sciatica such as routine exercise to strengthen muscles and also maintaining appropriate body posture in any way times.

The lumbar nerve roots originate from the spine and at the time they're susceptible to impingement out of a disk prolapse, inducing compression or inflammation of the nerve and also the signs of sciatica. Sciatic leg pain isn't common, affecting 3 to 5 percent of adults along with both genders equally. Men tend to be more inclined to receive it inside their 40s and ladies in their 50s, together with pain symptoms lasting more than 6 weeks in up to a quarter of cases. Physiotherapists are routinely requested to oversee the administration of sciatica.

When the intervertebral disk material prolapses, it induces injury by 2 mechanisms: direct mechanical compression of this nerve and chemical aggravation. The disk material shouldn't be outside the disk and its particular toxic compounds help swelling the neural as well as its surrounding structures, leading to congestion of the flow and also of their guts's ordinary message conduction. As the prolapse accounts for that sciatica it hasn't yet been demonstrated that the larger the prolapse the more acute anyone's pain.

The fantastic forces that we inflict on the minimal back imply the thoracic intervertebral disks suffer structural alterations along with prolapses. Many tasks involve a substantial degree of grip, such as bending over, performing motions in a vertical posture and lifting the arms apart from your system. This greatly magnifies the forces onto the disks and because of their fluid mechanisms that they suffer 3 5 times the heaps on the manhood. This could create the disk walls to bluff, providing feeble locations and predisposing to prolapse at a while.

The onset of lumbosacral radiculopathy can be surprising with low backpain along with some other spine pain can disappear at the onset of leg pain. Worsening facets are coughing, coughing and sitting together with bending or taking a stand common easing facet. Sciatic pain generally happens from the buttock back or side of their calf and leg and to the foot. In case the disk prolapse is high up (prolapses at disk degrees 11 to 13 are 5 percent of their total) the pain could possibly take the front part of the thigh no more compared to the knee. An individual might have a isolated field of pain but have a prolapse.

The physiotherapist will choose the individual's history with special awareness of "warning flag" which are signs of a severe medical reason behind the spine pain and the affected person won't be suitable to get physio. Weight loss, fever, night sweats, age (under 20 or more 55), issues with bowel and bladder control, acute beyond health background and also nighttime pain is going to be noticed. Any doubt implies citizenship to a health care provider for analysis. The physio will see some postural abnormalities and also the disposition, activity and position response of these pain signs.

A patient with spinal radiculopathy might display strange posture, sometimes flexed forwards and not able to bend backward, with a one-piece trunk change. Physiotherapists assess the capacity to do spinal motions, any pattern of restriction or trend for the annoyance to centralize on perennial moves. Physios can examine the springs, sensibility and muscular capability to carry out the neural examination. This and also the right leg raising test allow the physio to assess which of their spinal nerves is very likely to be to blame.

Discogenic pain may vary with recurrent motions, dispersing further towards the leg in towards the spine, the latter being termed as centralization. Physiotherapists utilize this happening to diagnose and cure disk related spine pain and also analyze the joints of the thoracic as knee and thigh pain might be known in an osteoarthritic hip joint. The complete history and examination eliminate patients who want medical referral for analysis and permit the physio to make cure plan.

Physio therapy laughter remedies incorporate many remedies: manipulation, mobilization procedure, lumbar equilibrium, myofascial discharge, McKenzie procedure (especially beneficial in disk prolapse), stabilizing massage, massage and soft tissue methods, painkillers, instruction of the individual, information on the ideal position to alleviate extreme aching pain along with remainder. Sciatica hastens as the inflammation and pressure simplicity however physiotherapists might suggest a continuous exercise plan to keep up straight back wellness over the very long run.

Most people today suffer with several diverse sorts of back pain and related back injuries, for example sciatica. When in pain, we all know to do is search out solutions. Broadly speaking we count upon a family practitioner or local clinical practitioner who we now have learned. This starts the individual at the "medical model" way of a settlement with the problem. Alas, the final effect for this particular version is frequently operation. Operation, even though sometimes necessary, is rarely the most effective alternative for first-time patients using sciatica. From another article we'll go over the positive aspects of chiropractic care to operation. It's going to tackle the good and the negative for both sorts of treatment.

The study discussed here has been ran with the national spine center at Alberta Canada and released in October of 2010 at the journal of manipulative and physiological therapeutics [inch]. The control group consisted of 40 patients who had been struggling with sciatica for longer than a couple of weeks. These patient's undergone treatments using pain drugs, making life style alterations, withstood physical therapy, failed massage or acupuncture without the consequences. Whenever these processes failed to work; their chief physician referred them to specialists which deemed them appropriate candidates for operation.

The people within this category were split in to two classes: one group experienced a medical procedure identified as microdiscectomy and one other type has been treated with a chiropractic utilizing conventional procedures. The patients got the ability of experiencing one other kind of treatment after a couple of weeks when these weren't pleased with the very first therapy.

What were the consequences?

The two groups saw noticeable improvements over baseline scores - significance which they watched noticeable improvements where as previous approaches had neglected. The complete 60 percent of the study participants profited from chiropractic spinal manipulation to the exact same level as though they failed operation. After 12 months there wasn't any difference in effect success dependent on the procedure technique. Which usually means that the total 60 percent of people called operation by their own primary care physicians and recognized as surgical applicants by the neuro surgeon might actually become similar results with chiropractic care. That will be a whole lot of potentially unnecessary anesthesia, cutting and er period. There's 1 paragraph from the results section with this study that's not hard to overlook, but exceptionally crucial. There have been originally 120 applicants which 60 met the study criteria and were asked to participate. Of those 60, 20 refused. Why? Because they'd not been given a substitute for operation; including as spinal manipulation. They did not desire to take part in the study and also be placed in the operation group without trying the spinal column manipulation! That really is incredibly telling. Not only does this demonstrate that there's still a demand for people and primary care physicians to learn about more regarding chiropractic processes, but in addition, it shows that folks comprehend the risks and costs of operation and would like to exhaust other possibilities.

This was that the initial study to look at those who'd neglected conventional medical direction of sciatica. Now many patients which neglect 'conservative maintenance' are known for a surgical test. We understand that 60 percent of those individuals can avoid surgery and have similar long-term effects together with acupuncture.

Sciatica has come to be the most commonplace back pain syndrome which affected millions of those mature people across the entire world. Cure for sciatica involves just proper straight back pain control. Sciatica treatments have come to be a multi-billion industry due to the expanding amount of men and women experiencing back pain. Physicians, nurses and other pros have gained advantage over offering the very best possible plan of treatment for relieving sciatica.

Treatments for sciatica demand traditional and non-conventional procedures. But people are now actually beginning to adopt the notion of choosing unconventional across the traditional treatments. With the existing uncertainty offered by a poor world economy, the seek out some other kinds of calculations revealed a radical increase through recent years. People today would like to come across a much cheaper and efficient method to put a stop with their unending struggle with plantar pain.

Ordinarily, direction for sciatica doesn't require to elect for extreme measures like operation and drugs, and unless there's a demand for you. Conservative kinds of treatments are consistently the first line of cure for sciatica. But appropriate identification of this inherent spinal illness stays the very best & most prosperous treatment in combating its outward symptoms. That really is being highlighted since burnout is a generally abbreviated symptom and also the most reasons the plan of treatment employed proves for a collapse. If you're some of the men and women who've tried virtually every treatment potential but still without a success, then a prognosis of the chief reason for sciatica is most probably undervalued.

Complete mattress remainder has become easily the most conservative approach that's ordinarily suggested by physician for being a cure for sciatica. Patients have been counseled to take short-term bed fractures in order for that pain to subside. Long term childbirth and protracted hospitalization are definitely frustrated. Deficiency of movement and also in activity could inflict more damage as a result of development of muscular corrosion. If your doctor happens to information more and protracted periods of bedrest, may too think about another most suitable choice.

Alternative treatments like chiropractic clinics, acupuncture and acupuncture are found to be a good method of treating sciatica. It has treatments and clinics that are much different from the standard treatments. It's obviously led by a professional or specialist such as for instance a certified therapist, acupressure pro and acupuncturist. They're the men and women who commence the treatment to make certain it's correctly handled.

CHAPTER SEVEN

❦

What to expect from pain management?

People frequently wrongly think about treatment by way of a pain management specialist as comprising just narcotic "painkillers "

But, the custom of pain medicine or pain control is identification driven only as with other healthcare specialties. As goes to a cardiologist to get a test of cardiovascular illness and receives treatment primarily based on a exceptional identification, a call into your pain management pro ends in unique treatment as every patient having pain is likewise different. The subject of pain medicine can be involved with the prevention, diagnosis, analysis, treatment, and treatment of debilitating ailments.

Infection affects more Americans compared to diabetes, cardiovascular problems and cancer combined. You can find approximately 116 million Americans with chronic pain, defined as pain that has lasted longer than three weeks and 25 million people who have severe pain.

Just like other physicians, the pain control pro should assess each affected individual and generate a plan for treatment on the basis of the individual's symptoms, examination and other findings. As an instance, the cardiologist must first examine you personally and create a few determinations. These generally include deciding if a cardiovascular illness will respond to fat reduction and exercise, if you've got elevated blood pressure and also want medication to reduce your blood pressure or if your cholesterol is either raised or if you own a congestion and desire an enhancement procedure or as a final resource, if you may possibly have to get called a coronary artery for coronary bypass operation.

All patients with coronary problems do not require the exact medications. This is contingent on the origin of the issue. Just because there are various treatments out there for cardiovascular problems, you can find certainly a huge quantity of treatment alternatives out there for orthopedic pain.

Even though patients may proceed into a pain management doctor because they "hurt," as they visit a cardiologist since all of them have heart issues, all pain doesn't reply to narcotics. It's a unfortunate and common offender when patients head to the pain management physician, they'll soon be treated with narcotics.

Treatments for spinal or spinal pain change like treatments for cardiovascular infection vary. It is dependent upon what's your explanation for your trouble.

First importantly, it's necessary to see there are several kinds of spinal or sinus pain. An individual may have muscle soreness, ligamentous pain, joint pain, bone pain, and distress as a result of herniated discs, pain by a fracture pain or pain by a pinched nerve or a nerve injury. Anxiety drugs are prescribed in relation to the resource of the painkillers.

Some patients that arrived at pain control never require pain medications. They can answer a ultrasound, additional intervention, bracing, or even into physical therapy. Our knowledge has grown into where we now know more how lousy posture and walking all perpetuate emotional pain. With complex utilization of exercises, tailored into someone's particulars demands, physical therapy could be helpful.

An test in physical therapy may possibly show that the individual's pain is due to lousy movement, tight muscles, rigid muscles, feeble musculature, or postural issues. As an instance, we are aware that patients with degenerative disc disorder, where the disc between 2 bones has begun to tear and wear, can reduce the pressure in the disc by exercising to boost your heart musculature and reduce or eliminate backpain.

Just like that the cardiologist who plays interventional procedures like coronary artery catheterizations, pain control physicians perform interventional approaches to reduce or eliminate pain, and operation as in different regions of medicine must be the final holiday season.

When you originally goto a cardiologist as a result of slight problem, i will be confident that a large part of you wouldn't ask"do i want surgery?" one wants to research different options before surgical interventions have been researched.

Out of experience, I've learned that patients perform best with treatment using way of a pain management specialist should they encounter with the exact same open mind and mindset at which they have been prepared to research a lot of options and become focused primarily on becoming narcotics or believing that operation is their sole alternative.

I used the illustration of this cardiologist because i understand that a large part folks might like that the cardiologist research all options before speaking us to a coronary artery. This is exactly the exact approach this someone ought to use while they've an ill or spinal issue. Always inquire about nonsurgical alternatives for the spinal or esophageal pain.

The pain management doctor, just like the cardiologist, doesn't function operation. Even the cardiologist does interventional methods, related medications, also manages your cardiac rehabilitation plan. Like wise a pain management doctor manages and sends your physical therapy or rehab application, prescribes medications, also plays interventional procedures. The two cardiologist and pain practitioner will probably consult with a physician if required.

Timing is essential to the results of one's treatment. You ought not delay a test for cardiovascular problems, nor if you proceed to discount spinal or spinal pain, and then wait overly long before trying a test having a pain specialist. I've seen too many patients wait too late during their treatment before looking for a pain specialist. As with other specialties, premature intervention could result in a better result.

Infection direction is a practice. It is made of numerous treatment plans and much more to the point, the remedy to the pain might well not be exactly the exact same since it really is for your own neighbor. Exactly enjoy a pacemaker could be the procedure of choice for the better half but maybe not the treating choice for you personally once you find that a cardiologist.

Innovations in pain-management

There has really been a wonderful shift in the life style of people who are in today's period, and people who have grown to be more prone to disease and illness. Anxiety is just one of those severe health problems that a lot of ailing men and women have. Anxiety can be painful, while it's actually a minor trauma or perhaps a life-threatening disease. There really are a range of trusted practices in U.S. who have produced innovative practices and remedies in managing pain. The indicators of pain could be alleviated with medications; however, medications have any unwanted effects. The growth and progress in technology have given rise to the invention of high level techniques and medications. The indicators of pain differ from one individual to another. It's dependent upon the individual's age, sex and physical stature. By working closely with the individual patient, a physician and pharmacist may prepare the suitable dose strength for extreme pain control.

Managing pain with drugs

Recognizing the idea of pain and its own control methods are shifting constantly. Various brand-new therapy plans are be-ings researched and introduced on an everyday basis. The most recent creations within the specialty of pain control would be of terrific value to the physicians in addition to professionals. A number of the qualities of latest processes contain achieving safe and durable relief systems that treat all sorts of human body aches. A number of the usual kinds of pains contain back pain, muscular, pain and pains related to illness or disease. For the majority of those pains, opioids having a prescription are regarded as effective on a momentary basis. Nevertheless, the opioid might decrease tolerance levels and also have any negative effects. Additionally, there are anti inflammatory and anti-inflammatory medications that have different negative effects, but are somewhat less habitforming.

Managing pain with remedies

There has become a excellent development in the specialty of pain control during treatments. Some of those advanced remedies that handle pain comprise celerel, painawaypro and therapize. These remedies expel the demand for narcotics. These treatments are utilized to take care of all types of pains which have neck pain back pain, postop pain and skin care conditions. The advanced remedies assist the individual in treating muscle strain in a simple way, regaining in less time, and increasing muscular strength.

Alternative pain management remedies

Additional studies have shown that conventional herbs may sometimes possess a long-term constructive effect, especially on arthritic painkillers. Included in these are the ingestion utilization of essential oils. Many essential oils possess pain and anti-inflammatory reducing properties if used frequently within a long-term using fewer side effects compared to many medication remedies. Consulting a naturopathic physician in combination with your doctor is preferred.

The two severe and chronic pain may interrupt your everyday living, especially with your leisure and work tasks. Perhaps this reason for pain is diagnosed or not, pain control methods may still help lots of people to no more suffer out of their ailment. In addition, it might permit the person to keep with their everyday tasks easily.

Infection is now turning into a significant problem within our society. In fact, nearly one third of the populace is afflicted by pain. Any pain is just one of the principal explanations for why individuals will proceed for appointment with their physician. Anxiety is a principal symptom in a lot of health circumstances, interfering with the standard of living and general functioning. If you're having pain on the human own body, don't just ignore it, thinking it will only go off. You won't ever know exactly what it's and it may just become worse should not assessed by your physician. This is the reason why pain control is a vital part of health since individuals forced to keep with the pain have a tendency to become miserable or using bad treatment benefits.

Earlier the ideal pain treatment therapy is given, health practitioners will determine the reason and also the kind of pain.

Mild pain essentially does occur immediately and may be mild or acute. However, it typically lasts just a brief moment. On the flip side, chronic pain is much more disagreeable and also the pain may endure during a long time period, hence impacting day to day living. Individuals afflicted by pain may experience an extremely thorough evaluation which includes their health background so the health care provider can completely understand the status and apply the ideal pain control treatment and technique.

Specialists on pain control utilize various kinds of processes which may efficiently suppress and minimize the disagreeable sensation. There are quite a few facets which can be considered ahead of the ideal pain control is provided. It features the spot where pain is situated, era of the average person, amount of physical limit and seriousness of pain.

Now, with the progress within the sphere of health, pain control techniques also have improved. The analyzed and recognized pain control methods comprise medications, injections, physical and rehabilitative services, disk compression, electric therapy treatment, back stimulation, neural racking processes and even comfort methods. Please be aware the patient ought to have a dynamic role in working together with health-related conditions as a way to relish long-term respite from pain. Besides that, behavioral interventions may radically enhance the life span of their individual, thereby reducing the recurrence of pain.

Infection is a symptom brought on by physical, emotional, or emotional injury or disease. At a certain point over time you should have observed pain no one understand that nobody is afflicted by afflicted disorders. You're a individual and everybody else you understand the very last time you've assessed and hence are vulnerable to annoyance. As this is actually the situation, you then must discover to take care of pain therefore you're able to alleviate the symptom to some bearable situation for a damaging patient or individual. That really is the pain control is about and also you also do not have to be described as a healthcare personnel to become in a position to handle pain to get some body. Even though some assert that working with anxiety is limited just to the physiological part, you should understand that helping some body may also enhance their emotional and psychological expectancy once they understand some one is taking care of them.

Caring is a part of human character so we'll spend money on your own normal tendency to nurture someone else in doing pain direction therefore you will possess the confidence to simply help someone minimize his bodily injury. You have to continue to keep this in mind whenever you're doing pain control in order for the patient is going to learn that you're attempting to help them whatsoever and they'll perform their job too. You have to have your head set your patient may get rude, irritable, and also repulsive of one's service however, you need to know they are simply byproducts of these pain and so they aren't personal in character. Taking good care of annoyance additionally involves a whole lot of emotional and mental efforts to help that you are equipped for the hard function as provider of pain control.

There are many sorts of aches one individual might consume therefore many procedures are hailed for various treatments for your pain. Bear in mind you can't really get rid of the foundation of physical strain but can only relieve it into pain control. You're fixing the symptoms rather than the true source of annoyance. There are lots of procedures for overall pain control and it'll soon be discussed briefly below. As a first rule, some pain felt from means of physician ought to be consulted together with his doctor or physician so you realize the reason for the vexation and you're able to assist the individual more efficiently.

Analgesics or medication made to help in alleviating pain are available in many varieties but caution medication needs to be observed. Medicine built to alleviate pain ought to be given at a pain squat, as advocated by who (world health organization). Pain ladder is traditionally employed as an overall principle in supplying drug for any kind of pain - this explains that the degree of pain and which sort of medicine is ideal for the problem. Mild pain ought to be treated with paracetamol or aspirin. Mild to moderate pain necessitates paracetamol having a combination with hydrocodone turns out to be a lot more effective. Moderate to severe pain is normally treated with more serious drugs such as morphine and identical medications with care because of their addictive side effects. Physical approach in relieving pain comes with acupuncture, tens (transcutaneous electric nerve stimulation) and physiatry. The majority of these procedures apply physical rehab and drugs. Bipolar strategy is based on emotional processes such as behavioral and cognitive therapy, biofeedback, and hypnosis to alleviate anxiety from emotional intervention.

Infection direction is 1 field of medicine that includes found several technological advancements all over the world. Spurred with this world wide phenomenon, chronic pain control practices in developing countries also have begun using innovative methods from the regions of pain killers, pain assessment, and intervention for chronic pain control.

Chronic pain may consult with any form of pain which suffers even with a personal accident was treated, pain associated with some degenerative or persistent disorder, long-term pain for the cause can't be diagnosed, or cancer disorder. Generally, pain which lasts even with half a year is chronic and takes treatment.

The identification and treatment of a specific patient in a chronic pain management practice usually demands the participation of several specialists including anesthesiologists, psychiatrists, physiatrists, neurologists, along with physicians and nurses. Several treatments are combined in sequence to make the individual feel comfortable when the pain can't be ceased, to help him/her come back to work, to get rid of their depression, and also to boost their bodily operation. Ergo, these remedies are drugs, operation, emotional counseling, therapies to excite the nerves, life style shifts, anesthesiologic treatments, and rehab.

Drug advocated for patients in chronic pain control practices may alter out of maids for pain that's not so awful to narcotic medication for more acute pain. Physical therapy is just one common therapeutic technique employed in the administration of chronic illness such practices. It involves training the affected person to boost his flexibility, endurance, endurance and potency; to relocate a means which is structurally safe and appropriate; & above all to manage pain. Therapeutic exercise can be a significant quality of physical therapy.

Still another crucial technique employed in chronic pain management practices is transcutaneous electric nerve stimulation (tens). This method offers aid to patients suffering from conditions like back pain or pain at the back, by the usage of non invasive household energy.

To amount up, once pain has been chronic, entire freedom from the pain will be not difficult. But, chronic pain control practices, throughout the usage of multiple methods utilized together with one another, helps sufferers of chronic pain like a fitter and more energetic lifestyle.

Infection management physicians ordinarily chance to be more anesthesiologists. Anesthesiologists make certain you're secure, weatherproof and comfortable throughout and after operation. Also they are at the office at the labour and delivery field, or at doctors' chambers at which debilitating tests or procedures have been performed. However, the processes employed by anesthesiologists have traveled outside these lands that are recognizable, also contributed to the evolution of a brand new kind of medicine called pain medication.

In many scenarios, an anesthesiologist directs a group of different physicians and specialists working together to ease your pain. The anesthesiologist or alternative pain medication physicians such as neurologists, oncologists, orthopedists, physiatrists and psychiatrists, and non-physician pros for example nurses, nurse practitioners, physician assistants, physical or rehab therapists and therapists, combine together to assess your problem. After an exhaustive appraisal, this group of pros develops a treatment plan for you personally.

Infection management physicians are pros at diagnosing the causes of the own pain in addition to curing the pain. Arthritis back and neck pain, cancer, pain, heart problems, migraines, shingles, along with phantom limb pain because of amputees are being among the most prevalent pain issues they generally manage.

Infection management physicians also treat severe pain brought on by operation, a painful disorder or even a significant accident. One of such pains is article knee joint replacement pain, headache during retrieval in the car collision, pain after chest or stomach operation, or pain related to sickle cell disorder. They could see to the patient at the clinic or at a hospital clinic.

The pain medication physician usually works closely together with your physician. They'll examine your medical records along with xrays as required. To get a very clear comprehension of the instance, they are going to provide you a thorough questionnaire. Your answers will enable them to assess the way your pain affects your everyday life. Pain management doctors may even perform a comprehensive physical exam on you personally. They could even select additional evaluations and examine all of the outcome to get the main cause of one's pain and also determine the way the situation may be solved.

No one likes to suffer with pain. A distressing sensation, pain can be really a result of the human anatomy to physical disease, trauma, or emotional illness. Pain is usually split into two types: acute and chronic. The former does occur unexpectedly as a result of trauma suffered by means of a tissue. The injury might be levied by whatever impacts human anatomy, i.e., operation, cancer or injury. Heartbeat and blood pressure usually increase in severe pain. However, when the reason for the pain is expunged, the pain normally goes off. Chronic pain, usually connected to some chronic illness, lasts more and there's a clear origin. Chronic lower back pain, chronic headaches, or cancer belongs to the category.

A pain management approach usually is contingent upon the character of this pain, i.e., if it's severe or chronic. Anxiety is usually handled by employing medical procedures, emotional procedures or other therapy approaches. In the instance of short-term severe pain due to an injury, normal medicines available on the counter, natural or herbal remedies and other medicines may be properly used. Chronic pain is much more difficult to handle, since it lasts longer and is much more technical.

Medi cal approaches might be broken to two chief techniques: medication treatment and operative intervention. Analgesic drugs may diminish or eliminate pain without affecting consciousness.

Psychotropic drugs act in the mind, affecting the individual's psychological condition. An individual should, nevertheless, be careful in their long-term consequences. Still another procedure used is neural wracking, in that a medication is injected round the proper guts to protect against the pain from reaching the mind.

The reason for the surgical branch of neural pathways is the fact that should the pathway has been cracked the pain cannot undergo. Even though maybe not operative at the authentic sense, transcutaneous electric nerve stimulation (tens) arouses skin area across the site of this pain together with the assistance of a power stimulator, also simplifies the aggravation messages using a tingling sensation.

Anybody, who's working with long-term or intense pain, also knows the "pain" from this illness. Typically, patients spend a significant period of time together with primary care health practitioners, physical therapist, and also pros, expecting to obtain a more permanent alternative. Interventional pain control is actually a practical alternative in such circumstances, where the patient has tried the other treatment choices.

Recognizing interventional pain control

Interventional pain management can be a technical field in medicine that addresses the identification and treatment for long-term or severe pain along with other associated disorders. This really is more of a "multidisciplinary" system, that will be extended by a group of experienced doctors and caregivers. With interventional pain control, medical PR actioners make an effort to reduce chronic and acute pain, besides emphasizing better living. The therapy is completely distinct from other kinds of pain control since there's not any direct dependence on pain-relief medications. Typically, your doctor may refer the issue to your pain management physician, who'll choose the degree of treatment, based upon the truth of this situation. In the event there is interventional pain control, pain management doctor will come with physicians, physical therapists, occupational therapists, therapists, neurologist, and orthopedic physician as needed to take care of the condition through the use of minimally invasive procedures like epidural injections, facet blocks, trigger point injections, etc.

Matters worth understanding

Interventional pain control is very good for patients that suffer from back and neck pain. Physicians can utilize more than 1 approach into the illness, based upon the identification. Using steroidal shots at the joints and also epidural space is quite common, whereas shots are also utilized to deal with a spinal nerve root, and this is recognized as the supply of annoyance killers. Branch cubes are also useful for diagnostic intention accompanied closely by radio frequency ablation, while health practitioners might also utilize extra shots from the side joints. Discography can be employed to obtain the potential source of pain, also within this particular procedure, a special dye can be employed within an injectable shape to some disk to know the pathology better.

In a few scenarios, minimally-invasive procedures such as"radio frequency ablation" could be properly used for its healthcare divisions, in order to confine the movement of nuisance signs. Doctors can also indicate using heated electrodes for many nerves which take the pain signs, which procedure can be understood as rhizotomy. Maybe not to forget, physical therapy and other kinds of occupational treatments are also employed for your own procedure. Doctors also indicate life style changes to patients, even should they find some other expectation to get much better health.

Along with as the health society is getting more keenly

conscious of the issue, physicians are thinking of regretting them. Therefore, a individual who has chronic back pain suffers, unless, their physician gets got the capability to refer these into a pain management center.

Referrals to a pain control Centre can be drawn up by almost any healthcare provider or an expert like a rheumatologist. Can this your physician passing the dollar because they don't really desire to bargain with you?

Perhaps not at all! If much of your maintenance or rheumatologist identifies one to a pain management center, it's in your own very best interest. A facility that's installed as interdisciplinary center, typically connected with hospitals or have an association with a medical college will have the ability to help handle your pain - free of restricted or no medicine

Because they truly are generally related to a hospital, so you can find medications like pain narcotics out there. However, they are going to initially make an effort to discover methods to handle your pain with no. What experts in those centers are finding is that too frequently, narcotics such as painkillers can give rise to a bunch of different issues.

The best way does all these facilities help?

Now you will be delegated to a group of pros. They'll examine the records that your main attention or rheumatologist sends them and they then are going to perform their very own preliminary assessments and analyzing. This might include blood workout, mris, x rays, etc.

Later they've this information gathered, the team will examine it and keep in touch with you regarding your history. What remedies or therapy you experienced and also how they worked or did not get the job done. You ought to be entirely fair and open with them around any portion of one's health history along with the way you live.

They will subsequently talk about this among themselves and generate a new plan which will be dealt with through the pain control center. You will assign to your chiropractor or physical therapist. You may possibly have meetings having a physiologist or psychologist. The team might believe you might take advantage of the massage therapist.

The goal of a pain control centre would be to exhaust other methods for managing the pain without narcotics. Sometimes, there'll be several medications prescribed in really tiny doses to get a while to workin combination with another remedies or remedies.

Exactly why the hesitation of medications?

A pain control center is dependent on what search has found. And research studies have discovered that people actually will undergo a rise in pain once they're on narcotics. Medication can alter how the body's immune system works. Endorphins are the organic painkiller. Granted there are people who are able to and can gain from narcotics, however also to automatically assume this could be the sole means to take care of pain would be an error.

Narcotic analgesics and opioids are very addictive to a patient. And there's also the concern of their interaction with other medications. For the ra patient, opioids won't cure their inflammation and also to get patients with fibromyalgia along with also the wide spread annoyance which is sold with, opioids just make it worse.

Later any operation, pain control is going to soon be important for both you and your physician. And if there's a degree of pain and distress to be likely after any sort of operation, your health care provider will require preventative measures to supply your ways to handle your pain. This is not just to continue to keep you comfortable, but if the own body is in distress, it cannot heal as fast as it will.

When you're just about to have surgery, your health care provider will go on your present medical wellbeing in addition to your health background. Always be fair and also notify them of any sort of medication you're taking, especially if you're already taking drugs to managing your own pain.

The kinds of pain to anticipate

Later operation, you might experience pain in regions which are going to be described as a surprise. Often times it's perhaps not at the operation website. Some regions where you may experience distress or pain following operation are:

- muscles - you might feel pain or distress in the field of one's spine, torso, chest, or shoulders. This stems from lying in 1 position on the table or the "tackling" the team may possibly perform together with you personally while at operation.
- throat - your neck may feel scratchy or tender. That really is from using any vibrations on your neck or mouth. Movement - any movement such as sitting or walking will probably soon be embarrassing and debilitating. Even coughing or coughing may cause greater pain.

Keeping your anxiety under control

Now you could have a significant role in your pain management by simply keeping your physician and the nursing team informed concerning your annoyance. Most of your will probably be quantified and through your hospital stay, you'll soon be asked to rate your pain on the scale with numbers zero through ten. Zero isn't any hassle and is the worst possible pain. This technique is effective for the healthcare team to discover how a pain control treatment is working or in case there's a requirement to create changes.

Who's may assist you to deal with your anxiety?

Now you as well as your health care provider will chat about your pain control before operation, deciding on what's acceptable for you personally. Sometimes doctors provide at a pain pro to work together with you after your operation.

At the very close of your day, even however, you're one which is likely to create the ultimate choice. Your health history and present health state is going to be employed by your physician and the pain pros to supply you the choices for pain control.

The various forms of pain management treatments

Additionally, it is more typical for an individual to be provided with more than 1 kind of pain control therapy. It's dependent on their wants and the sort of operation they'd had. Your physician and the pain specialist will probably create sure they're safe but effective, however, there's some amount of danger for any kind of drug. A number of the most widely used pain control therapies are:

- **intravenous pca (patient-controlled analgesia)**

Pca is a pump that's automatic and allows the individual to jelling safe levels of pain medication. The machine is programmed and can just release a particular amount within a particular period of time.

- **nerve blocks**

A nerve block controls pain in small, remote parts of the human anatomy. This system of pain control might be spread through an epidural catheter for protracted pain control.

- **cosmetic dentistry medications**

Later operation sooner or later, your physician will probably dictate some kind of pain control medication that's taken orally. You need to allow the nursing staff understand once you're having pain and when it's been over the typical four-hour interval, they provide you with precisely the prescribed dose.

Infection direction without drugs

There are tactics to attain pain control too. Such as directed imagery, a concentrated comfort method is effective by the individual' creating composed and tranquil pictures within their own mind. This emotional escape can also be enriched by hearing music and changing rankings.

Your physician might provide you guidelines for heat and cold therapy. This will diminish your pain and also some other swelling you might well be experiencing. For operation in the chest or abdominal area, employing a pillow for those who personally a cough, sneeze or simply take deep breaths can help being a process of pain control.

One of the best medical problems we frequently face in our day to day life is annoyance. As stated by estimation one-third individuals of earth are confronting issues of pain. Anxiety in just about any one of its kind vastly affects our own life quality. Pain management could be the name of a interdisciplinary approach which re-lives or helps in alleviating pain.

Infection management has distinct methods determined by the kind and potency of pain. In a given pain control team you can find after actors demanded. All these are medical professionals, clinical psychologists, physiotherapists, occupational therapists, nurses and pros etc.

Infection is very painful following a operation notably in orthopedic surgeries pain is sometimes described as an excellent problem for the patient since he could be totally on bed for a few of months. For that reason, pain control is essential for all these patients. Pain management can be necessary like an individual or patient afflicted the pain for quite a while will probably soon be a simple prey for melancholy which is likely to cause his life harder.

Infection is undesirable in its own kind and ought to be suitably handled for easy livings. There are lots of methods available that may assist in tackling the pain. This we shall mostly take in to consideration the pain control methods after a operation.

A pain management strategy after a operation can be multi disciplinary plus it may possibly be united with the input of healthcare professionals, acupuncturists, physiotherapists, chiropractors, clinical therapists and psychologists.

Most pain management methods after operation are dedicated to shared strategies and methods. Listed here are a few methods that actually help control pain after operations are after. Comfort is exceptionally useful feature in pain control and this system patient has been introduced to a relaxed and friendly atmosphere due to their physical and psychological comfort.

Deep breathing, progressive muscular relaxation (PMR) and fanciful gaudiness is useful for comfort. Exercises can also be also utilized to deal with pain after operation. These exercises are extremely simple bodily pursuits. Cold and heat treatments and stress direction can be utilized in several pain control systems.

Infection management may also involve any type of narcotics.

If pain after operation is immense simply than narcotics might be prescribed as narcotics take some side effects together with them which often leads the patient at a challenge if practiced at a standard routine.

Therapies may play vital part in pm (pain control) after operation. Massage can be of assistance to relax the muscle throughout the area of operation plus it'll lower the odds of redness and swelling in operation location. Emotional pain control methods may be practiced to take care of pain after operation. In this respect a proficient psychologist can also be hired which will coordinate together with patient and certainly will bring realistic consequences helping throughout the pm.

Food can be vital in discharging pain. For effective pm after operation an individual need to need to take care concerning the intakes of the patient because they matter. Some hypersensitive attack could occur with a few patients when their food isn't given precisely according to exactly what prescribed by a health care provider.

In case the pain is recurrence following the operation in relation to morphine may be supplied to the individual patient. Morphine is an important chemical in opium that's extremely effective against pain alleviation. It acts on the central nervous system of this patient also can be most widely used medicine for host pain after having a surgical operation. Morphine may be utilized to decrease pain such as chronic pain such as cancer. Tens machines may be employed for pm after having a operation. These machines also give a temporary pain relief in most people but those machines should really be just used with utmost caution.

Pairing chronic pain and storing it under control can be difficult. Most patients aren't certain about the total procedure and way of pain control, which explains the reason why they usually rely upon painkillers and medications for fast relief. In this informative article, we'll discuss pain control and matters which matter the most.

The basics

Chronic pain could be related to numerous illnesses, not limited by gout, unsuspected accidents, cancer treatment, and several other old and unhealed harms. When you've got persistent pain in another of one's own body parts for at least a month which does not appear to improve, you need to think about seeing a pain management physician. There are certainly a large selection of alternatives available, and typically, doctors often rely upon multiple treatments, based on the truth of this situation.

Recognizing pain better

Infection is real, and it may impact various individuals in an alternative way. To get example, when a certain patient is miserable about chronic pain, then his sense and emotional condition will probably differ from somebody else, who's suffered an unexpected harm. The entire process of pain control relies on several criteria. First things first, the doctor will think about the possible requirement for additional evaluation and identification. That can be essential for determining the entire nature and degree of treatment. He may also propose a couple of first items and lifestyle changes, in order to know the answer of this individual. When the pain is overly intense, he might also offer you extra drugs to reduce the inflammation, whilst to lower the total disquiet.